Sex with the Lights On

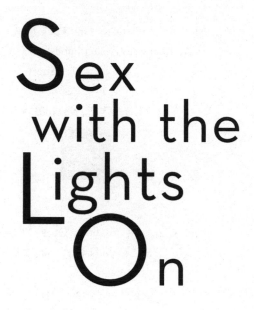

Sex with the Lights On

200
Illuminating
Sex Questions
Answered

by Ducky DooLittle

CARROLL & GRAF PUBLISHERS
NEW YORK

SEX WITH THE LIGHTS ON

Carroll & Graf Publishers
An Imprint of Avalon Publishing Group, Inc.
245 West 17th Street
11th Floor
New York, NY 10011

Copyright © 2006 by Ducky DooLittle
First Carroll & Graf edition 2006

Library of Congress Cataloging-in-Publication Data is available.

ISBN-10: 0-78671-680-0
ISBN-13: 978-0-78671-680-7

Printed in the United States of America
Interior design by Maria E. Torres
Distributed by Publishers Group West

for T. DOG

Author's Note

The health information presented in this book is meant for general purposes only and is not intended as a substitute for consultation with your physician or other health care professional. The materials presented are not intended as medical advice for individual problems. If you think you have a medical problem or symptom, please consult a qualified physician.

Contents

19. Butt Sex: Bottoms Up • 204

Acknowledgments

Thank You.

To my editor, Don Weise, for the wealth of insight, advice, and encouragement you have shared with me as we built this book together. I am very grateful for every ounce of kindness, wisdom, and patience you have given me. And thank you to everyone at Carroll & Graf and Avalon Publishing Group for all of your hard work and for simply having faith in me.

To photographer David Rodgers and makeup artist Jennifer Vega. Thank you for creating and capturing such beautiful images, including the photo on the cover of this book.

To my lawyer, Quinn Heraty, for all your advice and how you help to make sure my ducks are all in a row.

Thank you to all the sex teachers and authors that have schooled me and inspired me over the years. Some of you are very valued friends and others I simply admire based on the work you have put out into the world. Including Douglas Abrams, Kim Airs, Hanne Blank,

Joani Blank, Violet Blue, Kate Bornstein, Boston Women's Health Book Collective, Gloria Brame, Susie Bright, Barbara Carrellas, Claire Cavanah, Rebecca Chalker, Mantak Chia, Betty Dodson, the Federation of Feminist Women's Health Center, Nancy Friday, Guerrilla Girls, Stacy Haines, Paul Joannides, Midori, Mistress Morgana, Inga Muscio, Lou Paget, Planned Parenthood, Carol Queen, Candida Royalle, Anne Semans, Felice Shays, Cory Silverberg, Tristan Taormino, Rachel Venning, Veronica Vera, Beverly Whipple, Cathy Winks, and Sheri Winston. With an extra special thank you to sexologist Dr. Annie Sprinkle who, when I was just a young sex worker, taught me that the best way to live life is free of shame. No one can give it to you if you don't take it.

To Claire Cavanah and Rachel Venning of Babeland for taking me under your beautiful wings. And to all the present and past sex educators on staff at Babeland. I love you. You have succeeded in building a safe place for people of every gender and sexual orientation to explore sex. What a beautiful oasis you have created in this world. Thank you for the years we spent together while I was on staff. Thank you for mentoring me and believing in me.

To two very inspiring women who have dedicated their lives to uplifting a new breed of sex educator: home party salespeople. Jennifer (and everyone at Athena's Home Novelties) and Charmaine (and everyone at For Your Pleasure), you are positive and powerfully charged forces in the world. It is a gift to be invited to support you and all of your sex educators in your mission. Thank you for the support you give me as well.

To each person who has attended my workshops. Especially the brave souls who have shared bits and pieces of themselves and asked the questions included in this book. You teach me as I teach you and together we perpetuate more pleasure for everyone. I hope I have inspired you as much as you inspire me.

To all the women who have invited me to be a part of your private parties to teach sex, be it a bachelorette party, a birthday party, or just a night of sex talk with your friends. Together, in your living rooms, loft spaces, and hotel rooms, we have created a true word-of-mouth, grassroots sex education movement. And had a lot of fun doing it!

To each person who has come out to my live shows and all the venues that have hosted my appearances, on the road and in New York City. And to my oodles of friends who have helped promote shows and let me sleep on your couches. You have all been so loyal over the years and watched me grow as a performer. You push me to do bigger and better things with my life.

To all of the bloggers on LiveJournal.com who have been sharing words with me for more than five years. Thank you for being so generous with your thoughts, feelings, personal experiences, and preferences. You have expanded this book and made it more accessible and beautiful. Your instant online feedback and words of support only egg me on. Please feel free to take credit for any success I may have.

To you, the person who is holding this book in her or his hands. I hope the bits of knowledge I have shared will enrich your life if even in the most simple ways. I hope you will look at this book as an action book. Take the information that applies to your body, life, and lover(s) and please do something fun with it!

To everyone at the veterinary office on my block. This book would have been done faster if you had not convinced me to adopt the puppy you rescued. I did not even know I wanted a dog, but the warmth he has brought into my life is indescribable. Thanks for all the little things you do to help me raise him well.

To my beloved friend, confidante, and driver Kristine. Thank you for all the late nights and long drives we have spent together while touring and teaching sex across the country. Your ability to see beauty and humor in every situation has brightened my days. I honestly could not have done it without you. I adore you and look forward to seeing where the road may take us next.

To Michelle Bergstrom, my friend of so many years. We have grown up together. Thanks for skimming my words so I do not look as dyslexic as I am. And doing it with such care.

To my friends Josh and his talented EvilConspiracies.com for building my Web site and all the years you have rescued it in a pinch when I code html like a monkey.

To my family. T-Roy, Daniel, Phyllis, Jonathan, Rachel, and Jesse. Thank you for simply loving me.

To my husband. This book would not exist without your support. Thanks for letting me test my theories on you. Giving me a safe place to grow and learn, sexually and otherwise. I am blessed to be able to spend each and every day with you. I love you more each day.

Introduction

Accidental Sex Educator, or the Story of Ducky DooLittle

I had never ever considered myself sexy. Which is why it was so strange that I responded to an ad in the *Village Voice:* "Wanted: Sexy women to do phone work. 18 and over. Limited nudity in a fun and safe environment."

Was I sexy? Barely. If you like *Barely Legal* maybe. At eighteen I was old enough. Had I ever been nude? Almost. Once I let a boy look at me completely nude. But the lights were out. I did allow him to open the curtains to get as much moonlight as the sky would give him. More than anything I was just plain desperate.

It was getting cold in New York City and I had a raging case of bronchitis and no winter coat. I needed some cash, and quick, so I answered the ad. I figured I would take the gamble and let someone else determine if I was sexy or not. And that day the manager at Show World decided that, despite my bronchial wheezing, I was. With a little time and a few nice tips I eventually found a way to be nude too.

I worked on Forty-second Street for about a year. Every day I unlaced my combat boots, stripped down to my panties, popped on a pair of high heels, and waited for someone to drop their gold tokens, slip me a tip, and tell me everything. I'd stand there in the all together, listening over the phones that joined our two little peepshow closets, and they let loose. Some men told me their deepest sex fantasies, some exposed their fetishes, some just wanted to see me touching myself through the dirty Plexiglas window. Some wanted me to watch them in action. Every one had a different request. There were thousands of men who stepped up to my glass box and bared their secrets, each dirty request as unique as the color of his skin, the pattern of his body hair, and the curve of his cock.

The privacy and relative anonymity of the peepshow experience made it possible for those guys to be very honest with me. Consequently every night I came to work excited at the possibility of what I might learn. My patrons opened my eyes and my workday encounters lit a spark of sexual curiosity that to this day can't be put out. I absolutely had to understand what drives men's preferences and I soon became obsessed with analyzing and comparing my daily experiences. I listened carefully. I recited their requests over in my mind. I watched the way they touched themselves. I noticed the consistency of their semen as it rolled down the window. It was an amazing experience. I'm happy to have done it—and equally happy that there was a two-ply layer of Plexiglas between us! That was the beginning of my real education.

As fascinating as each day could be on Forty-second Street, I found that like most sex workers I had a limited amount of patience. Working in the sex industry is like any service industry: if you stay too long you get burned out. After I worked the peepshows, I stripped in clubs all over the tristate area. I did a brief stint as a dominatrix. Later I was a fetish model. I was a nudie magazine model as well.

Eventually I realized I needed a job where the size of my brain was at least as important as the size of my boobs. So I started writing for porn magazines. At first I had to promise each editor I would do a nudie photo layout to go with the words I wrote. But with a little time, the quality of my writing began to hold as much weight as my bra, and I became a full-fledged "sex journalist." My job as a journalist had me exploring sex in a whole new way—examining my own fantasies, interviewing hundreds of people on sexual technique, visiting sex parties, interviewing fetishists, and so on!

I began writing for culture and fashion magazines and started appearing on television shows as a "sexpert." People were incredibly responsive to what I had to say and I liked sharing my knowledge. I'd hear things like, "You are so bright and funny! And you really know what you are talking about." This was the beginning of my career as a sex educator.

In my private life I worked hard to gain as many sex skills as I could. I played the field, had sex in weird places, with weird people and weird objects. My tag line was "Hey, do you want to learn about sex from the guy who read about it in an academic book or from the woman who went out and screwed her way to getting your answer!" Everyone has been very responsive to the woman who went out and screwed!

For years I've kept my boat afloat by writing and performing on stages around the country. On stage I did burlesque and stand-up comedy. All of my comedy by the way was laced with smart sex messages, like how to avoid having to go to the emergency room with a potato stuck up your butt or how a guy can have more profound orgasms if he exercises his pelvic muscles by bouncing his hard cock like a low rider. (It's true!)

I also took a job at Babeland, a sex toy shop that prides itself in having quality products and even higher quality sex educators behind the counter. When it comes to expanding my sex knowledge, that was the real cherry on top. I spent long hours at Babeland, cataloging dildos, restocking condoms, consuming books, watching videos, and answers hundreds upon hundreds of sex questions. Eventually I became their lead workshop facilitator and the Education Coordinator of Babeland University.

Beyond the amplitude of my life experience, I have been trained in comprehensive safer sex by Planned Parenthood, attended Dr. Ruth's lectures at New York University, and—my biggest accomplishment—became an emergency room Rape Crisis and Domestic Violence Counselor in New York City.

Ask Me Anything

Little did I know when I answered that ad in the *Village Voice* that seventeen years later I would be teaching women and men all over the world how to amplify their sex play.

I find myself in big cities, small towns, and on campuses—it could be a room of ten or as many as two thousand people. I teach medical students, college students, social workers, moms, dads, church groups, gynecologists, movie stars, and professional athletes. Individuals of every gender and sexual orientation. The full scope of age, race, culture, and religion. I have a lot of answers, but I cannot possibly have the answer for every question as it applies to every individual. In those cases, my audience schools me. We grow together.

I start and end every workshop by telling my audience, "Ask me anything!" I urge them on by giving them blank index cards so they can ask their questions anonymously. This way the brave and the not-so-brave have equal opportunity to participate.

I have always opened up my presentations with index cards because I loathe the idea of getting up in front of a group of people and telling them what to do. It's not my style. Instead I inspire. I give options. I flirt with them and talk about all the possibilities that are available to us as sexual beings! And I do this with as many people as I possibly can.

These index cards have allowed me to teach people what they want to know. With their guidance I am not some blabbering head up in front of them, I am also a listener. I open up the conversation safely, and by the end of the workshop I have the whole room talking, sharing, educating and learning.

I must have been channeling that famed workaholic/sexaholic Alfred E. Kinsey as I meticulously filed the index cards away after each workshop. Over the years the thousands of cards started to speak to me. I loved the honesty each card possessed, a little piece of each person I had met. I even loved the handwriting. I had a private relationship with every index card in my collection.

It was not until my publisher asked me to write a book that I fully realized the rich value in these cards. I decided to write a book with help from the thousands of people I had met, been inspired by, and taught over the years—every question an actual question from someone out there. Were you one of them?

You Are a Sex Educator Too!

Even though this book is for everyone, not everything in it will be for you. Perhaps you think anal sex sounds painful. Or possibly I am writing about straight sex and you are lesbian? No matter what the topic, please stay with me. Read on. Absorb it. You may find one day that you need information that may not interest you at this very moment. If it does not apply to you, it may apply to your best friend, cousin, or child at some point.

Speaking of which, parents are the most important sex educators out there. But most studies show parents do not have the facts they need to teach their children effectively. For example, did you know that the Centers for Disease Control and Prevention reports that one in four sexually active teens will become infected with a sexually transmitted disease before receiving their high school diploma? Come on, moms and dads. Gain the knowledge, confidence, and language around sexuality so your children won't have to get their information from somewhere else. Because when they do, most often they are learning from their friends, the Internet, or pornography. Yikes!

Language

In live shows I vacillate between using the words *pussy* and *vagina*. (*Pussy* is my favorite word, but I have learned to also use *vagina* because when I make television and radio appearances I have to use words that won't get me thrown off the air!) No matter which word I use during speaking engagements it is very possible that I will see someone in the room actually flinch or laugh. They may not be used to hearing a person use more hardcore language. Or at least not in public. Perhaps they feel the word *pussy* is profane. At the same time the word *vagina* may offend the person next to them, finding that word to be too clinical or medical. Not sexy. We have no common language around sexuality.

Other times there will be people in the room with entirely different pronunciations for words like clitoris. One person will say "cli-*tor*-is," while the person next to them says "*clit*-oris." Maybe they have only ever read the word and never had to say it out loud.

These are just two of the many language observations I have made while teaching sex. We have plenty of words to describe our body parts and sex acts but not enough opportunities to use them! As you read this book, please don't let my language stop you from hearing my message.

Gender Is Fluid

For the most part I am defining gender in common male/female terms. But gender is not as simple as our English pronouns suggest. While most people feel cemented and confident in their gender, there are lots of people who are not simply male or female.

Some of us were born *intersex,* having anatomy that does not match the clear-cut definitions of male or female anatomy. In this instance we may have one ovary and one testicle, or anatomy that may appear externally male but be internally female or any variety of anatomical combinations. Many intersex individuals are surgically assigned a gender at birth or their parents chose a gender and raised their children accordingly. Sometimes intersex features surface only when an individual reaches puberty. Although some intersex people live pretty comfortably with their assignment, others find that nature and preference force them to define for themselves who they really are. Ultimately, gender is always self-defined.

Other gender variations include being *transsexual*. Many transsexuals feel an undeniable inner conflict with their biological sex. They may choose to go on hormone therapy and to have surgical reassignment or not. Transsexuality can occur in persons who were raised female but identify as a male (female to male—FTM) and in persons who were raised male but identify as a female (male to female—MTF).

You may also meet and fall in love with other *gender benders,* including *drag kings* (women who wear male clothing in everyday situations, in performance, for sexual pleasure, and/or as a political statement), *drag kings* (men who wear in female clothing in performance, for sexual pleasure, and/or as a political statement), *crossdressers* (women or men who live full-time or part-time in gender-defiant clothing), or any individual who refuses to be confined by gender stereotypes, be it through body, clothing, pronouns, politics, or sex. The individual who lives in that body defines her/his own gender labels. Keep your mind and your definitions open.

For the most part I use male and female pronouns, but when you see me refer to "all genders" you can be sure that I do this purposely. Gender is not limited to male and female but is full of amazing variations. If you have a lover who is gender variant, just as with any lover, you will need to ask that person to help you define where she/he finds pleasure.

Voices in This Book

The questions in this book are real questions, from real people. Just as the individuals who are quoted within this book are people who share the same online blog space with me. They so generously poured out their deepest secrets, true experiences, and bits of sex advice. I am very grateful to them because their voices have expanded the book immensely. I quoted them word for word.

Their contributions are funny, honest, sweet, and raw. Some of these people have been interacting with me online since I created my website nearly a decade ago. My online friends and fans are primarily female but also include a wide range of gender and orientation. (A special shout out to the guys on my blog space who, with a little gentle prodding, shared some very deep sexual secrets.)

This sex-positive online community we have built has been a cooperative effort of people linking to my site, people signing up for my E-mail newsletter at live shows and word of mouth. I hope you have as much fun soaking up their contributions as we had compiling them.

Please log on to my website www.duckydoolittle.com and join in the fun.

Love,
Ducky DooLittle

Anatomy

P leasure anatomy is much simpler than the world would lead you to believe. It's also more accessible than the 'here you will find the fallopian tube' anatomy lessons most of us received in health class.

There are no secrets to pleasure anatomy. The only secrets that exist are the ones you will find while exploring the unique ways of how and why you or your lover respond to particular touches, strokes, licks, smut, or toys! These secrets lie within you. Once you understand pleasure anatomy, unearthing your sexual possibilities becomes much more fun and easy!

I'll keep this anatomy lesson as nonclinical as possible. I am in no way trying to dumb things down; I am simply trying to sex everything up! Obviously when you're in a sexed-up frenzy there's no need to remember how to pronounce *pubococcygeus* (pew-bo-cock-sigh-gee-us) *muscles* when you could just say *muscles*. I'm here to lay down the necessary information to make it easy for you to find any part of your pleasure anatomy, understand its purpose, and ultimately tell your lover how to drive you wild with it!

HOMEWORK:

As you read about your pleasure anatomy, follow along!

1) Take off all your clothes.

2) Use pillows to prop yourself up in a comfortable position.

3) Use another pillow between your legs to prop up a hand mirror.

4) Use a flashlight and your fingers to follow along.

5) Look at the beauty of your body. Explore.

6) Use your hands to explore (spread your pussy lips or cup your balls) and watch how your body changes as you get sexually excited. Some spots might swell with excitement. Other areas might become flush with color. Very cool!

Looking at your own body in a mirror might sound hokey, but it is an important thing to do. A lot of us have never *really* looked at our own bodies. Not only is it interesting to explore your body, it is also good for your health. Knowing what your body looks like in a healthy state will help if you develop an infection or other medical problem.

Pussy:
Top to Bottom

A woman's external anatomy is called her vulva. Or if you are sassy like me you might call it pussy! Meow.

The first thing many women say when they see an illustration or photo of a pussy is, "Hey! I don't think my pussy looks like that!" Good. It shouldn't. No two pussies are alike and that is how it is supposed to be.

Some women have inner lips that are larger than their outer lips, many women have lips on each side of differing length or thickness, and some women have no inner lips at all. While some women have a nice, thick amount of what I call bumper, or fatty tissue in their lips and on their *pubic mound*, others have very little. The color variations are spectacular and, for many women, can deepen as one becomes sexually excited. This is natural, normal, and beautiful.

Pussies, like any other part of the anatomy, would not be nearly so interesting if they all looked the same. Although it would be impossible to share all the incredible varieties of shape, color, and size, I've included illustrations as merely a guide. With that in mind, don't look at any image of a pussy—be it the illustrations in this book, photos in a magazine, or women in adult films—and compare your body (or your lover's body) to the images you see. Doing this can lead to feelings of inferiority or even shame.

You have a pussy? Congratulations! It's beautiful.

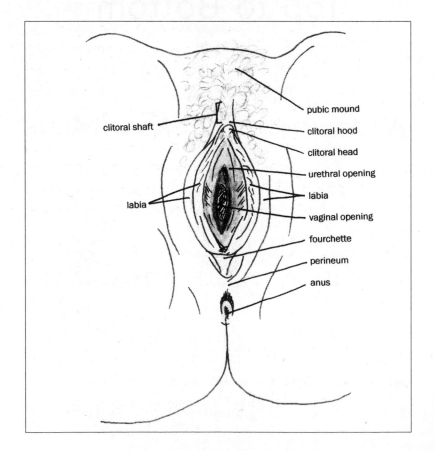

Her pussy begins with the *pubic mound* and ends with her *perineum* (Pronounced *"pear-"*—like the fruit—*"a-nee-um"*).

The pubic mound is easy. It's the padding that covers the pubic bone. It is fatty tissue that acts as a bumper during hot and heavy bouts of sex. It is easy to see because it is covered in protective pubic hair. As it rounds over the pubic bone toward the vaginal opening, the tissue has more blood vessels and erectile tissue and is far more sensitive to touch. Sometimes the pubic mound is called the *mons veneris,* which is Latin for "Mountain of Venus" (Venus being the Roman goddess of love and beauty, so that sounds about right).

Her *labia,* or lips, as they are commonly called, are the next most obvious feature. For most women there is an inner set and an outer set that make up her unique folds of skin. The size, shape, and color vary from woman to woman.

The outer lips have hair on them. For some women the outer lips may not be pronounced but sort of blend in with the skin of her inner thighs. However, for other women these lips are more juicy and obvious. The inner lips are usually hairless and more sensitive because the outer lips protect them.

A woman's lips can be very responsive to touch, tongues, or even a little hot breath! As a woman becomes aroused the blood vessels in her labia become engorged. The whole area will become flushed with color and swell with excitement. For some women this response is very apparent and for others it is much more subtle. When not a part of your sex play, the labia simply serve to protect her vaginal opening.

Where is the clitoris?

At the top of the lips where the two sides come together with her pubic mound, you will find the *clitoral hood*. It is exactly what it sounds like, a little hood of skin that comes down over *clitoral head*. The clitoral hood protects her clitoris. If she's into it, you can pull her clitoral hood back (toward her belly button) and expose her clit while going down on her or even just to see her clitoral head. Sometimes just using your fingers to tug at her clitoral hood can be enough to get a woman very aroused. Just ask her!

What is the average length of the clitoris?

The visible portion of the clit may be so small that it is barely visible, or it could be a full inch in length. The clitoral head and shaft is about one inch long on the average woman. The size of her clitoral head and shaft has no effect on her response. She may have a large clit that has minimal response or a small clit that is highly responsive. It's all relative to her unique response.

FACT:

In 1824 French doctors documented the case of a woman with a five-inch clitoral head. They reported that her clit was so large that at times it impeded her ability to have intercourse.

Depending upon the size of her clitoral head, you may or may not be able to see it. If it is elusive, gently pull the clitoral hood back toward her navel and the round little clitoral head will be apparent.

If you find yourself with a new lover, always approach her clit with the gentlest touch. You might even start just by cupping your hand over her entire vulva, then gauging her response. Once you have her in your hands, move your hand slowly. As she gets more excited you might ask her if she wants more direct clit stimulation. I say to do this slowly and gently because her clit can be very sensitive. It houses the thousands of nerve endings that are protected by the clitoral hood, ultimately making it the center of the universe.

That's right, the *Center of the Universe!* Or at least *her* pleasure universe. Never underestimate the power of the clit. It is the orgasm nerve center for almost every woman you will ever meet, making the clitoral head just the tip of the iceberg!

Yet throughout history, the clit has been underestimated. You may hear people refer to it as a "pearl" or a "pee-sized" organ. But more modern research by the Federation of Feminist Women's Health Centers and other scientists has found that the clit starts with the head, spans back toward the navel for about an inch (what we call the *shaft*), divides off into two *clitoral legs* that turn down to create a wishbone-like shape. These sensitive-to-the-touch clitoral legs sit under the lips, reaching three or so inches down from the clitoral head and shaft, ending near the vaginal opening with two bundles of firm tissue called the *bulbs of the vestibule.*

The clitoral legs sit above the pelvic muscles, but under the lips. In my workshops I tell women where these legs are and how responsive they are by reminding them how much fun they may have had as a young girl humping on "stuff." Stuff being a hand, a pillow, or perhaps even a stuffed animal! Some young women need a more solid surface like the rounded edge of table. (If this is you, be careful,

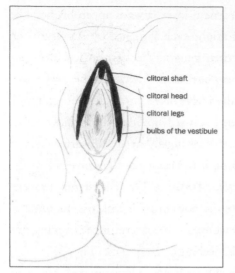

clitoral shaft

clitoral head

clitoral legs

bulbs of the vestibule

as excessive humping on hard surfaces can cause bruising or even bleeding. Take good care of yourself.)

Many girls grow up exploring this external region of their body long before they have any penetrative play. When young women get to the point where they start heavy petting with partners, they kick their heavy petting pleasure up a notch to include their partner's hand, leg, lap, and possibly that wonderful bump in their partner's jeans. This sort of play is all about a woman's clit and clitoral legs. And so you know: heavy petting is super hot at any age or level of experience. If you have not done it in a while, I suggest you give it a try.

While stimulating the clitoral legs and lips can be a ton of fun, orgasms are more often sparked by sensations applied directly on or very close to the clitoral head. I say "very close to" because some women are so sensitive that they like touch to happen near and around but not directly on their clit. Your partner is the only one that can tell you how and where exactly to touch her. The better you understand her body, the hotter your sex play will be.

During sex play you may find her clitoral head swells. At other moments it may seem to subside even though she is very excited. Like much of her pleasure anatomy, the area around the clitoral head is full of blood vessels and erectile tissue. This tissue can become so engorged that it sort of swallows up her clitoral head. All of this is normal and you shouldn't be concerned if at times you feel like you are playing now-you-see-it, now-you-don't with her clit.

Since women's bodies vary so widely, there's no one answer or simple answer to what will get your new partner off. You may have had a great touch that drove your last lover over the edge. Try it on your new lover and her reaction may be more like, "Whatever." Discovering what drives your partner wild will be a learning experience that, if you are lucky, evolves as long as the two of you are open to exploring together.

With that in mind, it is good to know right from the start that there are women who will not be into clit sensation. That's just the way nature made them. These women may be far too sensitive for you to touch them. They may be deeply connected to some other sensation like vaginal or anal play. In very few cases they may even have a damaged clit.

A damaged clit is usually caused by an accident of some kind. She may have fallen off her bike as a girl or hurt herself on a balance beam during gymnastics class. Any number of trauma to her pelvis might have caused damage. Frequently I hear from women who have had pelvic trauma as children who tell me their mom, dad, or doctor just did not want to talk much about it for fear of making them feel worse or embarrassing them. There is no shame in having had an accident like this or of any other kind. These women can go on to have super-hot and satisfying sex by tuning in to and developing other areas of their pleasure anatomy.

Typically what happens with trauma around the clitoral area is the body will develop scar tissue in the area where the trauma occurred.

This tissue can block access to the bundles of nerves that make up the clitoris. In more extreme cases the nerves can actually be severed and cause a complete loss of sensation in the clit. If you or your partner has had pelvic trauma, fear not, as you read on in this and upcoming chapters I will explain a number of other ways you may be able to bring yourself or your partner to orgasm that may not require clitoral stimulation.

HOMEWORK:

Female genital mutilation (FGM) is the custom of removing a young girl's clitoris, inner lips, and other sensitive bits. These surgeries are being performed in many cultures around the world, but mainly in countries in Africa and the Middle East. Why do some cultures mutilate girls? To control their sexuality. They believe that if a woman is mutilated it will cut down her desire for sex and the risk of her finding sex outside of her marriage. In these communities a woman who has not been mutilated is unmarriageable. According to Amnesty International, six thousand girls are mutilated every day, with the world's population of mutilated women a staggering 135 million. Worse, these surgeries are often conducted in nonsterile environments, putting girls at risk for infection, hemorrhaging, HIV, and death. You can log on to amnesty.org and participate in simple letter-writing campaigns to bring awareness to and stop FGM and other acts of violence against women.

Right below the clitoral head and between her inner lips is the *urethral opening*. Next to the clit, the urethral opening may not sound very glamorous but it is directly related to the much sought-after g-spot (another pleasure center for many women), so stay with me here!

The urethral opening can be hidden in the folds of her lips, very close to the *vaginal opening* or right at the opening. The urethral opening looks like a small slit and may be difficult to locate. It's actually a little hole that is the outlet for a two-inch tube connected to the bladder. This is where a woman's pee exits her body. If you did not know exactly where pee comes out of the female body, don't worry, lots of people don't know.

Because the urethral opening is so close to her vaginal opening it is vulnerable to bacterial infections, sometimes called urinary tract infections, or UTIs. This is an infection that starts in the urethra and can spread up into the bladder and ultimately the kidneys. It works like this: bacteria from her body or her lover's body (hands, penis, sex toys, butt) can get pushed up into this little opening during sex play and cause infection. I recommend that women go pee immediately after sex (not just intercourse, but any sex play where her vagina is touched) just to flush out the urethra. It's a bit of a hassle to run to the bathroom after sex, but if this little tip can save her the pain and expense of fighting a urinary tract infection it is well worth it.

A select number of women will find that stimulating the urethral

FACT:

The soft inner lips, urethra, and vaginal opening together are called the *vestibule* of the vagina. Vestibule means "entrance."

opening can feel good. I am not one to argue with where and how a woman finds her pleasure, but if you are experiencing repeated urinary tract infections I would avoid stimulating your urethral opening.

The vaginal opening is pretty simple. It is not the open tube that's often depicted in anatomy illustrations. The vaginal opening is more of a slit, with moist inner walls that actually touch each other. For some girls and young women, the vaginal opening can be almost completely closed off by a thin membrane of tissue called the *hymen.*

What is a hymen?

It is a membrane of tissue that many young girls and women have stretching across the vaginal opening. The average hymen is about one-twentieth to one-tenth of an inch thick. Some women are born with a hymen that blocks the vaginal opening almost entirely while other women are born with a very small amount of hymen.

A woman's hymen is typically torn the first time she has penetrative sex with a partner or alone if she inserts her finger or another object into her vagina. It can also be broken if she uses tampons, during a gynecological exam, or while participating in activities like riding a bike or other sports. When this happens she may experience a considerable amount of bleeding or so little that she does not even know it has happened. For some women their hymen tissue is very minute and/or elastic and breaks only if and when they give birth to a child.

As you look at the opening of a woman's vagina you may be able to see remnants of her hymen, depending upon how much tissue she had in the first place. These remnants will look like little tabs of skin.

MYTH:

In some societies and cultures where a woman is expected to be a virgin on her wedding night, her new husband will look at the bedsheets after she has sex for proof of blood, a sign that her hymen has been torn. For some cultures the wedding is not valid if the bride has not bled. This proves to be an incredibly unrealistic expectation for any woman to live up to, especially if she has a minimal amount of hymen or if her hymen is broken prior to her marriage. Desperate to make sure she meets this requirement, some women have been know to attempt to schedule their wedding around the time of their period, or to smuggle blood into the bedroom on their wedding night.

True Tales of Lost Hymens:

"I broke my hymen the first time I was fingered by someone else. I had fingered myself before that, but I guess either my fingers were not as big or I didn't do it as hard. It felt good and we didn't notice it until he had taken out his fingers and we saw blood on them."

"I lost my hymen the first time I used a tampon. I was fourteen and still a virgin. It hurt dizzyingly and almost scared me off of tampons completely. But I got over the fear!"

> **"**I was looking forward to a break, something inter-esting, painful—anything—but I guess it must have broken when I was young. I did karate for many years, and all the high kicks must have done it. **"**

"I believe it broke when I first used a sex toy, a big dildo, when I first managed to get it in all the way I felt something odd and there was a bit of blood. . . . I do not remember actually seeing it intact beforehand, so can't be sure."

"My hymen didn't break until one day when I was having sex with my third lover. He was really, really big, and the first couple of times I had sex with him were really painful. The time my hymen broke, I was just too turned on to care and we were at a hotel and I was on top and loud and something snapped and then it was much easier and felt better, and when I got up, I noticed blood."

"During my first penis-in-vagina experience there was bleeding. But I was so tired of being a virgin (I was twenty-one) that I told my very sweet, concerned boyfriend to keep going, even though I was in obvious pain. I just didn't care that it hurt. And after that, we didn't have penis-in-vagina sex again; my body stored that memory and just clamped my poor little vaginal muscles down anytime the penis came near. Even all these years later (now that I'm more of a size queen), my body still clamps down if a lover tries too much too soon."

"I actually tried to break my own hymen while masturbating with a vibrator. No go. The thing was impenetrable. When I finally had penis/vagina sex at age fourteen, my poor boyfriend managed to push into me and I yelped, shoved him away, and cried and bled for several days."

"I broke mine while I was masturbating. I stuck a hot dog in a condom and deflowered myself!"

At the lower side of the vaginal opening you will see a U-shaped band of skin. This is called the *fourchette*. This bit of skin is the tissue that connects a woman's inner and/or outer lips together at the bottom of her vulva.

What is the perineum and where is it located?

It is the section of strong skin, muscle, and tissue that separates the vulva from the anus. Guys have a perineum too. On a male it is the section of strong skin, muscle, and tissue that separates his balls from his anus.

If light pressure is applied just under a woman's fourchette, she will feel the strength of her *perineum*. Simply put, it separates her pussy from her *anus*. Because there are eight muscles all coming together at the perineum and some erectile tissue, many people enjoy it if they experience pressure, thumping, or vibration in this area. If you have never tried putting some pressure or a vibrator right on the perineum, I highly recommend giving it a try!

3.

Vagina:
Let's Go Deeper

S oft, warm, wet—the vagina is perfect in every way! This very elastic and muscular orifice will envelope almost anything you choose to slip inside there. The average vagina is about four inches from the vestibule to the cervix, but its ability to expand is incredible. A few women's vaginas will expand to twice their size when aroused.

The first one-third of the vaginal opening is loaded with nerve endings and very sensitive to touch, massage, and pressure. The deeper two-thirds curves slightly toward her navel and tends to be more responsive to fullness that comes with size and thrusting.

A woman's wetness will vary. Some vaginas are almost constantly wet, while others produce very little fluids. It is always a mistake to use the level of wetness to gauge how sexually excited a woman is or is not. She can be totally hot to trot and not be wet at all. Or vice versa.

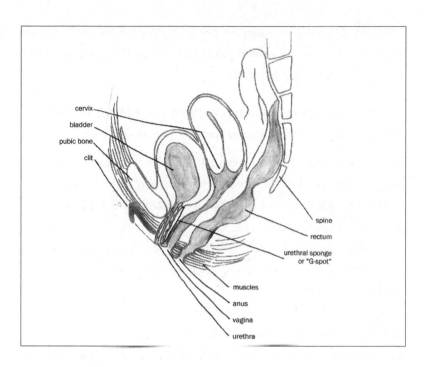

She may be wetter . . .
- if she is sexually excited
- while she is ovulating
- during different stages of her pregnancy

She may be less wet . . .
- the week or so after her period
- due to medications she may be taking
- if she is lactating
- after menopause

Either way, you should always keep a bottle of quality lube on hand to make sex play easier on her body. With lube you can have longer, hotter bouts of sex without the irritations that can come from all that hot and heavy friction!

I have a beautiful vagina but a short vaginal canal. How do I let a potential lover know before we have sex?

Say to your lover, "I have a beautiful but short vaginal canal." Just like you told me! But do it when the timing is right. Sometimes a person will feel more vulnerable about talking about the technical details of sex while naked. Or maybe you feel like blurting out, "I have a shallow vaginal canal." will interrupt the heat of the moment. For these reasons I recommend talking about specific needs before you ever get naked.

If you feel like you are ready to have sex with your lover, make a dinner date with your intention. Talk about your body's limitations, safer sex, and STD tests. Mix up the conversations so you can also include the flirty-dirty side of sex. Tell your partner about a fantasy you have or a position you have always wanted to try! Believe me, when you are sitting at dinner talking about the details of what kind of sex you like, your lover is only going to get more excited with the anticipation of what is to come. This is also a chance for your partner to share his or her sex needs and preferences, too. Once you are naked, you will be able to relax and enjoy yourself rather than worrying about how to get what you need.

Why is it that sometimes during sex with my guy he will hit the back of my vagina and I get a sharp pain?

Oh I hate that! That sharp pain can be enough to stop your sex play and make you wonder if you should be calling your doctor. But don't panic. He's most likely just bumping your cervix.

Your *cervix* is the amazing organ at the back of your vagina. It opens up into your uterus. It is the source of most of your vaginal fluids, including the alkaline secretions that clean your vagina and protect it from infection, the slippery wetness that lubricates sex and your menstrual fluids. If you use a speculum to look at your cervix, it looks like a firm round bump, not unlike the tip of your nose. If you have had a child, it may be larger, like the tip of your chin.

Some women love the feeling of having their cervix bumped during penetrative play. Other women hate it. Whether you are a lover or a hater of cervix bumping, you may find that around the time you are ovulating (about a week before your period) your cervix is more sensitive because it drops down a bit. If you feel that sharp pain, try to find a position where you partner delivers a shallower stroke or concentrate on sex play that is not about vaginal penetration. If you feel like the pain is more than just part of your monthly cycle, then you may want to see a doctor and check it out.

The vagina is the focus of so much of our attention. Most of the world mistakenly believes that sex starts with vaginal penetration and ends with orgasm. But don't let that narrow idea limit your sexual possibilities. Sex is about lips, eyes, hands, inner thighs, nipples, necks, and so much more! When you think about the vagina, look at it as an area that is loaded with sensation but also as a doorway to access other pleasurable parts of her deeper anatomy. Like her g-spot!

4.

G-spot:
Truth or Myth?

The g-spot is not a myth. I have found mine and I have personally found the g-spots of numerous other women. While the g-spot is a very interesting bit of female anatomy, don't get carried away with the hype. It is true that some women do find great pleasure in this area, but it's not true for every woman.

What is my g-spot and where is it?

The g-spot is an area that can bring surges of pleasure and inspire orgasms for some women. The g-spot is directly related to the *urethra*. The urethra is the short tube that is connected to a woman's bladder and allows pee to exit her body. The g-spot is the erectile and glandular tissue that surrounds the urethra. Sometimes it is referred to as the *urethral sponge*.

Contrary to what you may have heard, it is not the size of a dime or the shape of an almond. It is not a button. It is simply the tissue that wraps around you're your urethra. It spans the length of your urethra, about two inches inside your vagina on the front wall.

Why is it called the "g-spot"?

Because scientists love to name things after themselves! In this case it was Ernst Grafenberg, a German gynecologist, who in the 1940s wrote and published articles on the erotic possibilities of the urethra.

When sexually excited, women have erections, too. The g-spot is part of a woman's erection. I have already outlined how there is erectile tissue within the vulva, particularly around the clit and perineum. One very important thing that people do not recognize about female pleasure anatomy is that women have as much erectile tissue as men.

It works like this: for the first six weeks after a fetus is conceived, it is neither male nor female. At about six weeks the hormones kick in and begin to define gender. We all start out with the same parts, but they develop into different organs. For example the reproductive organs can grow into ovaries or testicles. The outer skin grows into labia or scrotum.

And for every gender there is erectile tissue that wraps around the urethra. For men this creates their very obvious penis shaft. In a similar way, women have erectile tissue wrapping their urethra. This spongy tissue is the g-spot.

Does everyone have a g-spot?

No. Only females have g-spots.

How do you find your g-spot?

If you are lying on your back, the g-spot is on the topside of your vagina—in other words on the navel side of your vaginal wall, under your pubic bone. It's not deep inside, but spanning the first couple of inches of the opening. It may be hard for you to find it with your fingers because it's in an awkward spot. You can try to prop your body up on pillow to make the search easier. You your can have a lover explore the area with his or her fingers or use a firm, curved sex toy.

You do not use a typical in and out motion but more of a focused massage. Ask your partner to insert two fingers about two knuckle deep and then push up and massage the top wall of your vagina.

If you are using a curved g-spotting sex toy, insert it about two inches with the curved tip pointed toward your top wall. Rather than working the toy in and out of your body, you should rock it up and down to create a nice, firm massaging motion.

If you do not feel a response immediately, keep going. Use your own hand or a vibrator to create some clitoral stimulation in conjunction with your g-spot massage. I know many women who have found amazing g-spot-centered orgasms with this technique!

What is the difference between a clitoris and a g-spot?

The clit and the g-spot are two areas that can bring on surges of pleasure for most women, but if you have never had a pleasure anatomy lesson (most people have not) they can be confusing. The basic difference is that the clit is stimulated primarily through the outside of a woman's body. The g-spot is stimulated inside, through her vaginal wall. The clit is on the top side of her pubic bone and the g-spot is on the underside. Stimulating the clit can get the g-spot excited and vice versa. Many women report clit stimulation as feeling very "nerve centered," while g-spot sensation feels more like a sensation of "fullness or intense pressure."

Is the g-spot in the same place for all women?

No. Yours may be at the top and center of your vagina or it could be a little bit to the left or right. But if you look in a mirror and find your urethra, you will get a good idea of where it is inside your body because your urethra runs parallel with your vagina.

Do you need to be turned on to feel your g-spot?

Yes. The urethral sponge becomes engorged as you become sexually excited. If you go searching around for it without being turned on you will have a hard time finding it or may feel a little irritation in your urethra. Many women report that once they are getting sexually excited (through penetration or clitoral stimulation), they will feel the corresponding tissue inside their vagina sort of pull together. Creating a slightly ridged area on the top wall of their vagina that feels something like the ridges on the roof of your mouth.

How do you know if you have found the g-spot?

For some women it will be very obvious. For others it is subtler. You start with a gentle but firm massage and if your g-spot is responsive the sensation may be immediate or it may slowly roll up on you.

I think I found my g-spot, but it was only OK—not mind-blowing. Was that really my g-spot?

For some women there is an instant and obvious reaction to g-spot stimulation. For others they may have no reaction at all or even find g-spot stimulation to be irritating. It's all about her body and its unique response.

I always compare sexual response (in the g-spot or any other hot spots) to our feet. Some people could plop down and fully enjoy a never-ending foot massage. Other people think a foot massage is no big deal. And then some people cannot bear having their feet even touched, much less massaged. This is how their body reacts to that kind of touch. The same is true for sexual response.

I have also had a number of women say they had no real g-spot sensation for most of their lives and then suddenly one day, with the right toy or the right partner their g-spot will become responsive.

The best you can do is explore, love your body, and focus the bulk of your attention on the areas of your body where you know you will find the best sensations.

What if you cannot find your g-spot?

For a lot of women their g-spot is not responsive. That is normal. If you have searched for it with your fingers, a toy and maybe a partner, and there is no response, then you are one of the normal people who have a nonresponsive g-spot. No big deal. Go back to where you find your pleasure, with your clit, muscles, partner, sex toy . . .

***

True Tales of G-spotting (Or Not):

"I'm 35 and I just found mine last year, with the help of a very sensitive, younger boyfriend. He was surprised when I told him it had never been stimulated previously. Neither I nor anyone else had taken much interest in finding it before."

"I have yet to find my g-spot, no matter how hard I try. My fingers are simply not long enough, toys don't seem to find it, and partners have not found it. I remember reading something in one of my mother's magazines when I was about ten about how the g-spot apparently does not really 'show' until you are older. It is probably just be myth of course, although could have some element of truth to it, as certainly in my experience sex gets better for women the older they get—maybe that is why. I am not too concerned about not being able to find it, although granted a little frustrated because I want to know what it is like!"

❝I remember once I started having sex that some positions would send little thrills along my belly. It wasn't consistent from lover to lover though. I don't remember when I heard about the g-spot and I did find an area that feels very similar to my soft palate generally where the g-spot is supposed to be but a little further in. Playing with it myself doesn't seem to do a lot—I get distracted by the texture and have to use odd angles to get my fingers there.**❞**

When being aroused with my g-spot, why do I feel like I have to pee?

Ah yes, the pee sensation. It is very common, but I can teach you how to stop that from happening to your body!

For most women the pee sensation is the beginning of g-spot

stimulation. I have already outlined how the urethra is part of our g-spot. When we are young we trained like puppies not to pee on stuff. When ever we get the slightest sensation in our urethra our body sends a signal to our brain that has us running to the lavatory. But guess what? During sex your urethra is not getting stimulated by a full bladder. Instead it is getting stimulated through your vaginal wall. You do not need to pee. Your nerves are just sending you a wrong signal.

It can be so distracting that you actually stop having sex, hop up and run to the bathroom! Once in the bathroom, you sit down on the toilet and suddenly you *can't go!* It's so frustrating.

Here's the deal. Your body is built to either have sex or go pee, but not do them at the same time! Part of the function of your urethral sponge is to swell up and close off your urethra. The same thing happens to men. When they have an erection they cannot go pee.

The next time you are having sex and you feel like you have to pee, try taking a deep breath and keep screwing. Do not stop having sex. Your body is not going to betray you. You are not going to pee the bed. Stay focused on your partner, your toy, your other senses. Do not let the pee sensation interrupt your sex play. For most women there is g-spot sensation on the other side of that pee sensation but they let the pee sensation derail them and they never get past it.

This will be frustrating the first few times you do it, but the more you do it the easier it will become. Essentially you are retraining your nerves and brain to recognize that during sex, that pee sensation does not mean you actually need to pee. Eventually you will stop feeling it all together.

5

Female Ejaculation: More Wet

When sexually excited, women may release an extra surge of fluid. This surge is sometimes referred to as *female ejaculation*. A woman's body can do this before she orgasms, while she is orgasming, or even after she orgasms. Ejaculating can feel like an intense spray of fluid or it can feel like a subtle change in wetness or friction. For this reason I believe *ejaculation* is the wrong term for what females do. I think using a term like *wet surge* would be more fitting, but people have adopted the other term to define this phenomenon, so I will just put the word in quotes.

Can all women ejaculate?

Yes. Every woman does produce this fluid. Simply put, it is the wet spot on the bed. (I apologize to all of you ladies who have been successfully blaming your partners for the wet spot! It is in fact us.)

Some women produce more of this fluid than others. Your "ejaculation" fluid may leave a significant wet spot on the bed or it may be
just a few droplets.

   You may feel yourself or your lover release this fluid when you are
having penetrative play and suddenly the friction changes. It will
feel like someone added a little water to your lube. That is her glandular fluid.

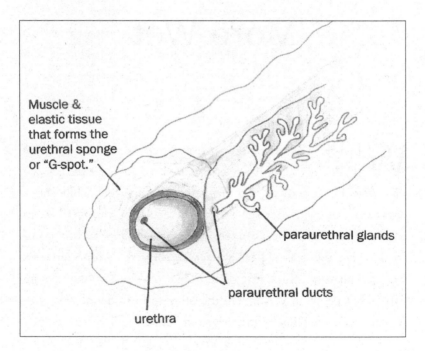

Muscle &
elastic tissue
that forms the
urethral sponge
or "G-spot."

paraurethral glands

paraurethral ducts

urethra

What is female ejaculate composed of?

If we take a closer look at the urethral sponge you can see that it is
loaded with *paraurethral glands*. These glands drain into the urethra
through little ducts. This fluid does come out of the urethra. For this
reason some classify it as purely pee and dismiss the entire subject. I

argue this point because although this fluid does drain out of the urethra it does not originate from the bladder.

What exactly this fluid is composed of is still, in my opinion, speculative. So few studies have been done on female pleasure anatomy that the bulk of knowledge I have comes from my own personal experience, the experiences of the many sex educators I have studied with, and from the thousands of workshop participants I have worked with over the years.

The two scientific female "ejaculation" studies I have come across include one, where they gave a number of women a digestible pill that turned their pee blue. When they had these women "ejaculate," the fluid that they released was not blue; at most, it had a slight blue tint.

In the other study they collected samples of this "ejaculatory" fluid from a number of women and compared it to the test subjects' urine. They found the fluid is glandular in nature with trace amounts of urine. The trace amounts of urine they attribute to the fact that the glandular fluid washes through the urethra and may collect any residual urine.

My personal experience has proven the fluid is clear, has no scent or a musky scent, and is salty. My own "ejaculatory" fluid reminds me of tears.

Why do some women squirt during orgasm and others do not?

"Ejaculation" is similar to g-spotting in that her body will have its own special way of responding to stimulation and expressing "ejaculation." To begin with, you may be a person who squirts before or after orgasm. That is normal.

This fluid can be released out of some women in dramatic, explosive spurt or series of spurts. But for most women it is squeezed out of her body in a less dramatic way. Sometimes the release is blocked by the toy or partner who may be penetrating her and simply dribbles out around them or flows out of her body when they pull out. This may be because her urethral opening is positioned closer to her vaginal opening or because the toy or position being used causes pressure against her urethral opening.

True Tales of Female Ejaculation:

"My girlfriend ejaculates pretty regularly when she climaxes, and pretty dramatically. She gets embarrassed about it sometimes, but I think it's great, as long as we remember to put down towels on the bed. In short, female ejaculation is great but sleeping in a puddle is not so great!"

"I have been ejaculated on. I think of it as a sign I'm doing something right—like getting extra bonus points on a video game."

"I don't know if I have ever done it. I certainly think every woman is perfectly capable of ejaculating. I am half convinced I probably have done it without even noticing."

"My boyfriend and I have a polyamorous relationship. The last two girlfriends we had were copious squirters. I can, too, but it takes hours to get enough internal stimulation for me, and I usually end up sore, but when I do, *wow!*"

"It has happened to me once. I was around nineteen years old. Not sure why it happened then and not since. It freaked me out. At first I thought I had peed, but it wasn't pee. I don't mind that I haven't ejaculated since that one time. It's not something that would make sex better to me. If you can, cool. If you can't, that's cool, too."

"I've never been able to ejaculate but several of my lovers can and it turns me on to no end. I've been trying for years without success. I can find and stimulate my g-spot and have g-spot orgasms but there's no ejaculation."

"I've found that my girlfriends who can do it, no matter how otherwise sexually liberated they are, are always somewhat embarrassed about it. They know what it is and recognize it as a positive thing but are still a little shy about it."

❝ I am a female ejaculator. When I was younger it didn't happen very often and I'd get really embarrassed when it did. I wasn't quite sure what was happening and I would instantly run away and hide. It didn't help that the guys I was with had a less than positive reaction to it. Then I dated a guy who absolutely loved it. He would have me ejaculate all over his face and chest and he loved every minute of it. That made me even more comfortable with it and like it even more. ❞

How do the women in adult films squirt so much liquid?

It is important that you never compare your body or your lover's body to the individuals you see in films. The women they hire have what I call "stunt pussies"! Just as they hire men with especially large penises, they will also hire women who have bodies that are usually extraordinary in one way or another.

So how do they squirt like that? It depends upon the woman. Some of them may have an especially large urethral sponge and/or increased capacity within their paraurethral glands. Other women have been known to fill their vagina with water and use their muscles to squirt it out. The producers will use creative editing to make movie magic happen. That's Hollywood for ya!

How can I learn to ejaculate?

The two most common factors that lead to ejaculation are firm g-spot stimulation and strong pelvic muscles. A nice deep massage of the g-spot (urethral sponge) can help it swell to an even larger size, and eventually you can use that massaging action to squeeze the fluid out of the urethral sponge.

If your muscles are strong enough they may be able to put enough force on the urethral sponge to squeeze the fluid out or it may happen uncontrollably during an orgasm. If you are actually attempting to "ejaculate," try bearing down with your muscles. You do need to have fairly strong pelvic muscles to make that happen, however. And even then, some women's bodies are just not built to "ejaculate." You'll learn more in the next chapter about female pelvic muscles and how to strengthen them.

Explore your body and see what it responds to. But if your body does not "ejaculate" in the manner you had hoped, don't despair. Just have fun trying!

I hate getting the bed wet. Is there any way I can stop myself from ejaculating?

When it comes to "ejaculation" I meet lots of women who believe the grass is greener on the other side. Some women are eager to learn how to "ejaculate." They feel like they are missing out on a special orgasm and get frustrated searching for that "golden 'gasm." On the other hand women who *do* get very wet are sometimes totally embarrassed by this. They feel as if they are losing control, even peeing during sex sometimes or find it embarrassing to wash the sheets after every bout of sex.

If you "ejaculate" with every (or almost every) play session but want to stay dry, the only advice I have is to go to your nearest pet supply store and buy puppy pads. These are absorbent pads with a plastic backing, built for sopping up fluids. Lay one on your bed before your get really hot and heavy. Or you can lay one on your mattress before you put your fitted sheet on to protect your mattress. These pads make no sound and no one will ever to know it is there.

Some Kind of Sex Monster

One of my first sexual experiences ended in disaster when I unexpectedly "ejaculated" on my lover. I was happily doing just what came naturally without an ounce of self-consciousness. I was on top of this young man, whom I had admired for some time, and in a mind-numbing state of excitement—complete with a racing heartbeat,

heavy breathing, and blurry vision. It suddenly became apparent that
my partner, however, did not seem to agree.

He jumped up in a panic, pushing me off, and declared that I had
peed on him! It all happened so quickly that I sat there stunned. My
heart dropped. I knew I had not peed. At least I thought I hadn't. I
mean, I knew what it felt like to pee and I had not felt that sensation. Sure, things were a little wet—and maybe because he had been
lying under me he was the wetter of the two of us, but what had just
happened?

Without another word he was off to the bathroom. I imagined he
was washing my wetness off of him. In the dim light of the bedroom
I put on my jewelry, got dressed, and slipped out the door. I left what
had been the most exciting sexual encounter I had ever had feeling
totally humiliated. I never saw him again.

That experience haunted me for years. I was hesitant to have
sex again. I felt like I could not control my body, like some kind
of unlovable sex monster. I wanted sex and had so much natural
desire, but I worried that any sexual encounter could end in
humiliation.

Eventually I shared my experience with a female friend, who
assured me that her body did the same thing. From there I found
a number of books that gave me a fuller understanding of female
sexual response. Ultimately I have encountered so many women
who have had similarly been baffled by their body's natural
response. Now, after seventeen years of research, I have met

countless individuals who embrace female "ejaculation" as a healthy and exciting sexual response.

Today I look back at that boy and feel sorry for him.

6.

Female Pelvic Muscles: Bigger, Better Orgasms!

The female pelvic muscles are totally underexplored and the fact that they are the force behind every orgasm is seldom recognized. The huge amount of hype centered on the g-spot and female "ejaculation" at the exclusion of all else frustrates me at times. Every woman has a g-spot, but not all g-spots produce the same sensation. Every woman produces "ejaculate," but most women do not spray it out during orgasm. The pelvic muscles are a different story! In terms of orgasmic possibilities, these muscles rank up there with the clitoris.

The stronger your pelvic muscles, the stronger your orgasms. It's that simple. (This is true for individuals of every gender.) When we orgasm these muscles contract involuntarily. The better aware you are of your pelvic muscles' location, how they work, and when to engage them, the easier it will be for you to manipulate your orgasm. For many of us this can lead to elongated orgasms and multiple orgasms.

FACT:

The dictionary definition of an orgasm is "the peak of sexual excitement, characterized by strong feelings of pleasure and by a series of involuntary contractions of the muscles of the genitals."

What are Kegels?

Arnold Kegel (pronounced "*kay*-gul") was a medical doctor who was very outspoken about the benefits of exercising the pelvic muscles. He helped women overcome urinary incontinence by instructing them in how to exercise their muscles. You may have heard how women who have recently given birth or are reaching the age of about fifty or sixty can have problems with incontinence (involuntary peeing). They might have a good laugh, coug, or sneeze and end up releasing a little bit of pee. If a woman keeps her muscles in good shape, there is far less chance that she will ever have that problem. Other problems that can arise from weak pelvic muscles include a prolapsed uterus. That's when a woman's uterus partially falls out of her body. (Not good.) These were the problems Dr. Kegel was dedicated to solving.

The exercises he designed proved to enhance orgasmic response as well and became known as Kegel exercises. Sometimes people refer to these muscles as the Kegel muscles.

You may also hear the Kegel muscles referred to as the pelvic muscles or the PC (pubococcygeus) muscles. These are three different names for the same set of muscles, which include the vaginal muscles, the urethral muscles (which stop and start the flow of pee), and the anal sphincter muscles. A total of eight muscles that all come together at the perineum.

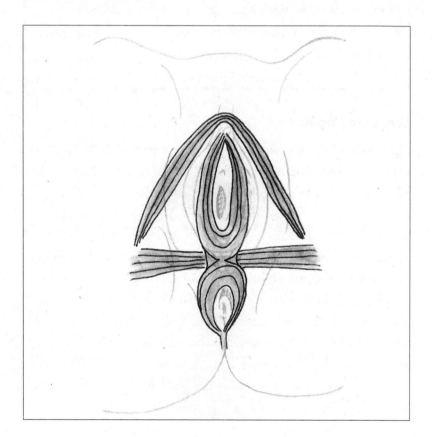

Healthy pelvic muscles are important for women to have for reasons beyond orgasms and the ability to start and stop the flow of pee. If a woman plans on ever having children, her strong muscles will make it easier for her to carry the baby, birth the baby, and ultimately heal from having the baby. Keep 'em strong!

I have heard that once a woman has a baby she is loose down there. Is this true?

The tissue that makes up the vaginal walls is more elastic than any other part of the human body. With a little bit of healing time the walls will spring back to their normal size. The muscle, however, can be traumatized, which might make your vagina feel loose. Muscle trauma can also affect a woman's body's ability to hold urine. She may leak a little pee if stress is applied to her abdomen. Exercising her pelvic muscles will not only stop the pee problems but tighten her vagina. However, in the rare cases where childbirth is especially traumatic, reconstructive surgery may be required.

If you are pregnant or have recently given birth be patient with your body. Sharing your body with a child through pregnancy and breast-feeding is a serious trip. You will have physical and emotional reactions to these experiences that may distort your sense of self and possibly your body image. Take time to care for yourself. If your lover has children, it's worth going out of your way to arrange for her/him to have solo rest time. Ultimately this will raise your lover's spirits, leave her/him feeling less stressed, with more energy—all of which can lead to more sex!

True Tales of Strong Muscles and Orgasms:

"The way I go into orgasm (after some stimulation already)

is by clamping down really hard on my PC muscles. One of the problems with having strong muscles is that my muscles will actually pull condoms off, but there's not much else to do except deal with it, because I virtually don't enjoy penetration without holding my PC muscles really tight."

"I've been a PC muscle flexer since I was a little girl. Long before I discovered the joys of clitoral stimulation, I'd flex those little pelvic muscles like a pre-masturbating fiend. I'd squeeze and squeeze them until I was afraid I'd pee my pants. These days, I don't make it a point to purposely work my pelvic muscles. I just naturally flex that stuff without thinking. And when I have an orgasm, there's definitely a lot of heavy-duty muscle spasms happening. In fact, my strongest orgasms tend to occur when I am clit-stimulated to peak and then penetrated forcefully. Having something push inside me while my muscles are flexing is an incredible sensation and can usually prolong my orgasm for several minutes. My lovers often remark how "strong" and "tight" my vagina feels. And while I love having a muscular pussy, it can also be a bit of an annoyance sometimes. I can't seem to keep things inside of me when I need to. Things like tampons, contraceptive sponges, dildos. One flex and I shoot them across the room!"

" About two years ago I attended a workshop Ducky did and she mentioned those muscles and how to exercise them. I thought I would give it a try and start doing a few Kegal exercises a day. Not too long ago I was on top of my partner when we thought we heard my son wake up in the other room. We stopped what we were doing to listen for a moment but I stayed on top with him still inside me. All of a sudden he asked me "What are you doing? That feels amazing!" I hadn't realized but I was tightening and letting go of my muscles. He just loved it and now has started asking me to do that more often. I never knew how much better sex could be when those muscles are toned. Thank you so much, Ducky! "

If these muscles are so wonderful, then why have I never heard of them?

Because they exist in the area of our bodies that the world perceives to be our "naughty bits." Our society is so sexually repressed that no one wants to talk honestly about anything having to do with our pelvic region. But they are muscles, as important as every other muscles in our body. Do the world a favor and tell everyone you know!

HOMEWORK:

Be a vaginal scientist. Use the information I have provided to explore your partner's vagina with your fingers and toys. Be scientific with your pleasure. Test pleasure theories and make notes about what you find. While you experiment, ask her yes-or-no questions. (It can be hard for her to talk when her brain is sexed up!) Try a deep-tissue massage in her g-spot area. Ask her to flex her muscles for you. With time and discipline she will become strong enough that you will be able to feel her muscles flex around your fingers. Use your other hand, a vibrator, or your warm breath on her clit and see what kinds of changes occur in her body. Her pussy might swell in excitement, change color; her breath might deepen, her muscles might flex, or her hips may rise up. If you are in for some role-playing, get a clipboard and a lab coat and play sex doctor!

How can a woman build strength in her pelvic muscles?

The sexiest way? Flex them rhythmically during solo play or partner play. With or without penetration, use your breath, muscle, and hip movements to create a rhythmic motion that moves through your body. As you breathe air into your lungs think about breathing air in through your pussy as well. Release and exhale at the same time. Just keep breathing and flexing until you feel dizzy. For most women this will result in a better orgasm right away and build strength at the same time.

There are also some great toys/tools that can do wonderful things for your muscles! There are a number of different high-grade metal barbells that are made for this purpose. They weigh about one pound. You lie down on your back, insert the toy/tool in your vagina, and flex around it. You are literally lifting weights with your pussy! For more fun you can masturbate with the barbell inside yourself. Many women love the smooth surface and cool metal sensation, plus solid metal can bring fantastic g-spot pleasure.

Smart Balls are also very effective. They are two attached silicone balls, about an inch and a half in circumference. Insert them in your vagina before going about your daily routine. (I do not recommend running errands with Smart Balls in your pussy because they may fall out and cause an uncomfortable situation for you and others.) They way they work is simple: by holding them inside you are clenching your muscles and exercising. A side note, they can also be fun to put inside your body while you use a vibrator on your clit.

For best results use these techniques in conjunction with these exercises.

How to Exercise Female Pelvic Muscles

For women, locating your muscles is easy. You use these muscles to stop the flow of pee. Clench your muscle right now as if you were trying to stop the flow of pee. Do you feel your pelvic muscles rise up? If not, you might try flexing this muscle once while you are actually peeing. Although it's OK to try this now to help locate your muscles, I do not recommend stopping the flow of pee if you do not have to. Doing so can cause reflux (urine going back up your urethra) and in some cases lead to urinary tract infections.

Make sure you focus directly on the pelvic floor muscles, not your stomach muscles or your upper thigh and butt muscles.

Once you have located your muscle I recommend doing these exercises immediately after you have peed because doing them is easier when your bladder is empty. Plus, doing them after each time you pee makes it easy to remember to do the exercise.

Since these muscles are internal and no one can see a

woman flex, some people say, "You can do these exercises any-where! On the bus, at a stoplight, or at your desk!" I recom-mend you do them in a place where you can concentrate and take deep breaths. You will get better, faster results this way.

These exercises can be annoying and frustrating when you first start doing them, but don't let that stop you. The more you work these muscles the easier the exercising becomes.

Follow these simple steps:

- Let all of the pee out of your body.
- Flex your muscles ten times. Think about squeezing out a sponge with your vagina. Do three sets, for a total of thirty flexes.
- Be sure to breathe deeply.
- Do this three times a day or every time you go pee.

Or

- Let all of the pee out of your body.
- Flex your muscles and hold for two to four seconds. Think about squeezing out a sponge with your vagina.
- Relax for ten seconds.
- Do ten sets.
- Be sure to breathe deeply.
- Do this three times a day or every time you go pee.

How I Accidentally Became Hyper-Orgasmic

I may sound like I am obsessed with the pelvic muscles but it's for good reason. Years before I was born my mother was in a bone-crushing, near fatal car accident. While suffering through the pain of learning how to walk again she developed a drug addiction that would haunt her the rest of her life. Part of this is because of me. My family speculates that her drug addiction later led to the birth defects. I was born with twisted bones in my legs that demanded heavy metal braces. As a toddler, I also had one lazy eye that required I be fitted for hyper-corrective glasses, which were made with just one prescription lens; the other lens was nonprescription. Consequently, when you looked me straight in the face my right, good eye looked normal while my left, bad eye looked *humongous.*

Between the braces and the giant eye I caused a real scene. Strangers would ask my mother in a loud voice, "Can she hear me!" As if my googly eye and miniature glasses had somehow made me deaf as well.

"Yup. I sure can," I would smartly reply and then wait for the laughter that followed. I did not know exactly why they were laughing but I loved laughing, too, so who cares. Right?

It only took a few years for those two birth defects to be corrected, but another problem was discovered when I was seven years old. After years of painful and extremely baffling kidney and bladder infections, the doctors found my urinary tract had not formed properly.

The numerous exploratory surgeries uncovered the source of the birth defect as well as how to repair the problem. They were not sure I would survive the surgeries, but they knew for certain that I would eventually die if they did not try.

I had thirteen surgeries in all. I spent a year in the hospital. One of the toughest parts of the hospitalization was the catheter they had inserted into my urethra.

If you do not know what a catheter is, it's a device that essentially pees for you. A tube was inserted into my urethra and into my bladder, allowing my pee to drain directly into a plastic pouch, which a nurse would carefully empty every now and then. This kept my bladder empty and reduced chances of infection. The catheter also meant that they did not have to disturb my aching body to get me to the bathroom day and night. Through all this I slowly healed, regained my strength, and finally they took the catheter out.

As if living with the catheter was not bad enough, what it did to my pelvic muscles was even worse. Because I did not have to pee on my own accord for so long, I was not using my pelvic muscles to hold my pee or to stop and start the flow of pee. My muscles became so weak from lack of use that I literally could no longer control them.

Pee would just drip from my body. It was horrible. I was not sophisticated enough to express my feelings at the time but I felt like my body was trying to betray me in every way possible.

But this is where it gets good!

There was a nurse at the hospital, an amazing, gentle woman, who sat me down and taught me how to exercise my pelvic muscles so that one day I could regain control of them.

Once I figured out exactly which muscles she was talking about, it was pretty easy. All I needed to do was take a few minutes to flex my muscles thirty times, three times a day, for a total of ninety flexes a day.

The nurse made me promise that I would do these exercises each and every day. She put such an emphasis on the value of these exercises that when I made that promise, like any seven-year-old would, I took it *very seriously.*

I went home and I did my pelvic muscles exercises. And I did them every day.

But the funny thing was that *no one ever told me to stop* doing my exercises. I only knew I had to do them every day or else I might die or pee or who knows what! So by the time I turned eight I had developed such strength in my pelvic muscles that I was orgasming just by flexing my muscles.

I had suddenly found pleasure in a part of my body that had brought me such extreme pain and embarrassment. Almost spontaneously this body that had betrayed me at every turn was making up for lost time. Although I had never heard the word masturbation and did not even know there was a name for it, suddenly I became totally obsessed with it. Ultimately, masturbating and orgasming only made my body stronger.

Today I can bring myself to orgasm simply by flexing my muscles and breathing. But don't be too impressed. I am not special. I don't have some kind of stunt pussy. I am just a perfect example of a person who came from a place of disability and in less than a year, through a little discipline, became incredibly orgasmic. If I could do it, then you can, too!

7

Chests, Breasts, & Nipples

Breasts are not just beautiful. For many people they are incredible nerve centers, too. For others they feel best when simply being admired and not touched.

What do normal breasts looks like? They can be small, big, full, flat, soft and solid. They can be similar in size or one breast may differ in size from the other. Areolas can be so light that you can barely see it or black as night. Nipples can be large, small, poke out, lay flat or invert. Many women whose breast grew fast or who have experienced pregnancy have stretch marks. For women they have little glandular bumps that surround the areola. Both men and women can have hair around the areolas. Breasts change in size with weight gain/lose and life cycles like menstruation, pregnancy and menopause. All of this is normal.

I hear about creams that can increase the size of breasts. Do these really work?

No. There are no creams that will enlarge your breasts. The healthiest way to improve your breast size and shape is to exercise your pectoral muscles though push-ups and weightlifting. Another great thing women can do for themselves is to stop comparing their size and shape (or your lover's size and shape) to that of others. You are beautiful. The more you believe that you are beautiful, the truer it becomes.

MYTH:

Many people mistakenly equate breast size with sexual appetite. Nor does breasts size govern how sensitive a person's breasts may or may not be.

It is also a myth that erect nipples indicate excitement. The truth is that a person's nipples can become erect for many reasons, including temperature changes, sensation or irritation from clothing, and sexual excitement.

FACT:

According to the American Academy of Family Physicians, 2 to 6 percent of humans have a third nipple.

My man loves boobs. Sometimes a little too much. How can I get him to be gentler?

Show him. Let him watch how you like to be touched. Letting a partner watch you touch yourself will drive almost anyone wild. If your partner is smart, he will see what you are doing and steal your moves! If your partner is touching you in a manner that is not enjoyable, let him know. But equally as import, when he is doing something right be sure to let him know that as well. Positive reinforcement in sex play is very powerful.

I know my girlfriend likes to have her breasts touched, but why is it that sometimes she will shy away from me?

The only person who can really answer that question is your girlfriend. Ask her.

For many women, their breasts will be swollen and sore a week or so before their period. Breasts that otherwise beg for attention may, at this time of the month, be too sensitive to touch. Or for other women, this is the time they really want extra breast attention.

Some of the large-breasted women I have spoken with have told me that too much sexual attention directed at their breasts can leave them feeling uncomfortable. You may want to direct attention toward your partner's chest that is not purely sexual in nature. By this I mean things like giving her a massage, including her shoulders, breasts, underarms, and ribs. Let her experience the massage with no pressure to have sex. This positive, nonsexual attention will have her feeling less objectified and more relaxed in your hands. Plus, it's a great way to get to know her body and possibly even screen for changes in her breasts that are signs of breast cancer.

Are inverted nipples sensitive to touch?

Absolutely. An inverted nipple is one that tucks inward rather than pointing out, but like any other nipple shape and size the sexual response is relative to the individual. One woman with inverted nipples may love to be touched while and some other woman with inverted nipples may hate it.

Do guys like to have their nipples licked and sucked?

Some definitely do! Others are totally hands, tongues, and teeth off. Ask him—or lick him and see how he responds. Just like with women, guys who respond well to nipple play find it can be a great source of arousal.

True Tales of Nipple Play:

"I'm an equal opportunity nipple girl. I love having mine played with as much as I enjoy teasing my partner's nipples."

"During foreplay/sex, yes. Any other time, no. If I'm not in a sexy mood, it's irritating."

"I used to like a lot of nipple stimulation (pulling, light clamping, biting, etc.), but I've been breast-feeding for the last two years, so right now my nipples are kind of burnt out by the time it's time for grown-up playtime."

"If I'm not already turned on, touching my nipples is not

going to do it, I'd rather they be left alone. But once I'm really excited, feeling my nipples pulled or pinched is often the thing that brings me to orgasm."

"I love having my nipples sucked, rubbed, or twisted. I like firm pressure, but nothing sharp. If I'm not already turned on, though, it's just irritating. I can also reach orgasm much more easily if my nipples are being manipulated at the same time as my clit—it feels like there's a little invisible string connecting them!"

"I find myself irritated with people grabbing my nipples. I only want them played with when I'm already turned on. If I am not already turned on, then it's just annoying."

❝ I love having my nipples touched and licked, with a little bit of pressure. I most enjoy it as 'multitasking,' and more readily achieve orgasm if a man is stimulating my nipples at the same time as oral, manual, or full penetration. ❞

"I'm not big into clamps, but a good tug can feel hot. As with pretty much everything sex, the more turned on I am, the more rough and intense you can get with them."

"I'm ridiculously oral, and when I had a tongue piercing it got rave reviews from several lovers when it came to using it on a nipple in conjunction with sucking. I think there's something about the firm pressure of the ball from the piercing."

"I'm a one-way nippler myself. I love to play with nipples, but I don't like mine messed with."

"For a many years I didn't think I was into anything nipple related. . . . It just didn't move me. And then . . . well, it turns out that my lovers were not being rough enough!"

"I'm for stroked, licked, caressed, gently squeezed, lightly tugged on, and lots of kissing and licking. Then once I hit a point I want them to be twisted, pulled, bitten, pinched, and generally handled roughly. The odd thing is that even though I try to explain it and will tell my lovers which I want (words ranging from 'gently' to 'bite!') there are some who cannot disassociate the harder play with the extreme passion that is necessary to do it. So they think that the hard play is a way to get the extreme passion and not something possible because of it. I can explain it again and again, but once it's wired into some people I can't seem to get them to stop biting when I want gentle. It's one of the ways I judge whether or not to keep a lover."

"Licked, stroked, sucked . . . yes. Pinched, twisted, pulled, clamped . . . *no!*"

"My nipples are not very sensitive, and I usually find it boring and/or irritating to have them messed with much. Except when I have PMS, and then they're more sensitive and hungrier for attention."

"Sucking on nipples is the best as far as I'm concerned. . . . I once came very close to having an orgasm just from that, with a lover who just focused on all the different techniques one can incorporate into sucking. It was heavenly."

8.

Penis:
Tip to Base

P enis, cock, dick, salami, cupid's ramrod or whatever you may choose to call it, the penis is monumental! Shapes can vary from long and thin to short and thick, to long and thick, to short and thin. An erect penis can poke out like a straight arrow, rise up like a galloping horse or point down to the ground. All of these shapes and sizes, in any combination, are normal and wonderful! Because we can see the penis and hold it in our hands, we tend to simplify this beautiful bit of anatomy, but read on and learn how complex and fascinating the penis really is.

FACT:

The word *penis* is the Latin term for tail.

The helmet shaped tip is a very sensitive area for most guys. This tip is called the *glans,* or head of the penis, and it is loaded with nerves. It is said that the head of the penis is about as sensitive as the sole of the foot, so every little touch will deliver amplified response.

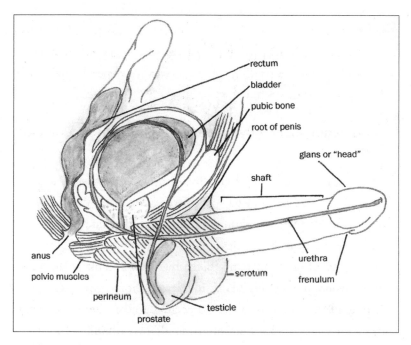

His head may or may not be covered by a sleeve of skin called *foreskin.* If he has foreskin, you can gently pull it back and see his full head. The foreskin will protect the nerve endings on the head of his penis. Once the foreskin is pulled back you'll find he may be more sensitive in this area than a guy who does not have foreskin.

The foreskin can be fun because once it is pulled back this sleeve of skin helps create stokes that are more fluid during a hand job, blowjob, or during penetration.

If he does not have foreskin, then he has been *circumcised.* Circumcision is a surgical procedure, most often performed while the male is still an infant, where the foreskin is removed. This surgery is common in the United States for newborns of all denominations, and worldwide for newborns of Jewish and Muslim descent.

A circumcised penis can be a bit more rough-and-tumble because the nerves on the head are not quite as sensitive as an uncircumcised penis. But as with everything sexual, it always depends upon that individual's response to touch.

I heard circumcised guys are cleaner than uncircumcised guys?

Traditionally people believed circumcision made it possible to keep the penis cleaner. That may have been true a thousand years ago, but studies show that with modern plumbing and hygiene practices this is no longer an issue.

At the tip of his head you will see his *urethra.* This is the small opening where pee and ejaculate are released. Some guys like sensation around their urethra while other guys find it irritating. You'll have to ask your guy if his urethra is hands-on or hands-off.

Which part of the penis is most sensitive?

Almost every guy agrees the *frenulum* area (under the head) is the hottest spot. This area is very responsive to the kind of licking and circling that can only be achieved with a warm, wet tongue or well-lubricated fingertips. The frenulum is on the under side of his head if he is standing up, where the ridge of his head come together at a point. This hot spot includes that point, over and around the ridge and where it meets the shaft. I have interviewed more than a thousand guys and almost every one of them told me this is the hottest spot on the penis.

As we move over the tip and down onto the *shaft*, the penis is made up of three parallel, spongy cylinders that together crate the shaft. The two cylinders that make up the top of his shaft have strong veins that run through them that are surrounded by tissue that make up tons of chambers. The cylinder on the bottom side of his shaft is made up of the same tissue but has his urethra running through the center of it.

When he is soft the chambers are empty and collapsed. When his nerves are stimulated the muscles that restrict the two veins relax and allow blood to rush into the chambers, filling the penis to capacity and causing an erection! Depending upon the color of his skin you may see his penis darken as he becomes erect.

These chambers can fill up very quickly or the process can happen in stages. How fast he gets an erection depends upon the person and can vary from day to day. Studies done by sexologist Alfred Kinsey found that erection speed is determined by many factors, such as fatigue, alcohol consumption, health, and the degree of arousal.

His erection will subside more slowly than it came on because the capillaries that allow the blood to flow out of his penis are very small.

When, why and where an erection happens can be very unpredictable. A touch or a thought might stimulates those nerves. Or it could be a sensation caused by his clothes rubbing him in a certain way. It is normal for some guys to get an erection when they least expect it. It is also normal for a guy to be unable to get an erection when he wants it most. This is just the mechanics of the human body.

> ## FACT:
>
> It is against the law for a man's erection to show through his clothes in Arizona, Florida, Idaho, Indiana, Massachusetts, Mississippi, Nebraska, Nevada, New York, Ohio, Oklahoma, Oregon, South Dakota, Tennessee, Utah, Vermont, Washington, D.C., and Wisconsin.

True Tales of Male Hot Spots and How to Touch Them:

"I like overall pressure on my shaft and head combined with smooth warm lubricated friction. Rhythm is everything."

" Wrapping your thumb and forefinger around the base or using a cock ring can increase the pressure, making it harder and more sensitive. You can pull in more pressure by milking with your hand, or sucking with your mouth. But there's a point where that hurts, so you might want to calibrate all of these sensations with your guy. **"**

"The most sensitive part is definitely the underside of the tip. On the head of the cock I like very light touches if there is no lubrication yet, but if it's wet I like a thumb and forefinger clasped in an O-shape to be rubbed around the tip. Along the shaft I like a nice firm grip from the base to the tip, then back down. It feels really amazing when someone starts at the base, strokes up, passes their open palm across the tip, then gets a good firm grip back on the shaft on the return trip back to the base. Lather, rinse, and repeat until he pops!"

"A very, very light caressing of the sides of the shaft with fingertips would be totally arousing, especially if I would happen to be tied up to the bed. This is a very hot way to tease a guy who is all tied up and can't go anywhere."

"If you don't know what to do, just ask us. We have had this cock our entire lives and we know just what we like when it comes to making it feel good. Not to say we're not into new forms of stimulation, but as I've said before an open dialogue will generally lead to better orgasms."

"The best spot is the underside, just below the head of my penis. Sometimes I can orgasm from just rubbing there with one finger. Also, the top edge of my head, the rim of it, is a big spot for arousal. Also, running a single finger up the underside of my shaft feels good. Grasping it with index and thumb in an O-shape and running just that up and down with pressure feels good. Grasping the entire shaft and moving the skin up and down where it curls over my head some feels good, too."

How long is the average penis hard and soft?

The average soft penis is 3.4 inches in length. The average erect penis is 5 inches. While these numbers can be interesting, I recommend never comparing your own body or your lover's body to averages, statistics, photos, or porn film stars. It's futile. The most important thing when it comes to male pleasure anatomy is not having a generous size but being sexually generous in a more broad sense.

MYTH:

Some people believe you can judge what size a guy's erection will be by looking at his size when he is flaccid. This is completely false. There is even the common locker room saying, "I'm a grower, not a show-er." Which means my cock may look small when it's soft but once it is hard I'm really *huge!*

Does size matter?

In my experience I find the person's mind, fingers, and mouth are as important as his penis. A lover with the biggest penis or no penis at all could have me a thousand different ways if they engaged my imagination and use everything they have to take me over the edge. Size is not important to me.

This is not true for everyone. Some people crave a large penis while others may, for any number of reasons, need a smaller one.

For a number of years I worked at a sex toy store called Babeland. One of the walls in the store was dedicated to nothing but dildos— lots and lots of colorful dildos in every shape and size. I do not know how many hours of my life I stood by that wall of dildos, helping customers find the right phallic toy for their body. Consequently I have had a *lot* of conversations about size.

The larger dildos, for the most part, were massed together on one side of the wall and the smaller ones at the other end. A customer would come in and see the largest dildo (a two-pound, nearly nine-inch Goliath called Spinal Tap) and ask, "Is that the largest dildo you have?" Our largest dildo would not be big enough to fit their needs. (So to speak!) While the next customer might come in and see the smallest dildo (a thin, four-incher called Silk) and ask, "Is that the smallest dildo you have?" Of course, this just proves that size is relative to the individual.

FACT:

According to a survey conducted by the *Village Voice,* when women were asked what they found most attractive in a man they said: 39 percent butt, 28 percent "other," 15 percent slimness, 11 percent eyes, 5 percent tallness, 2 percent penis. Now you know, guys. It's your ass that gets the most attention! If you really want to grab the attention of women maybe you should walk backward!

How do you make sex with a small penis feel good for a woman?

You can start by recognizing that sex is much bigger than intercourse. Great sex includes flirting, kissing, oral sex, fingers, sex toys, penetration, and imagination. Great sex happens when each partner is as interested in seeing their partner get off as they are in getting off themselves. Tune in to your lover, listen to her breath, watch her hips moves, feel her muscles flex around your fingers. Talk to her honestly about how she likes to be touched. Encourage her to touch herself, watch what she does and steal her moves. Read great sex books and pick up new techniques. Read erotica to her in bed. I could go on and on. Great sex has little to do with penis size. And if you do by chance fall in love with a Size Queen, buy her the biggest dildo she can handle, sit back, and enjoy the show!

How to Enlarge Your Penis (Or Not)

1) Lose weight. It is estimated that, for every thirty-five pounds of weight gained, a man loses one inch in penis length because the body fat creates padding around the base of his penis.

2) Surgery. You can legitimately add up to two inches in length by cutting two ligaments in your pelvis. (Ouch.) In a separate surgery you can add considerable amounts of girth by inject fat from your belly or butt into your penis. Although the girth surgeries have proven to be less effective because the body will often reabsorb that fat in as little as a year after surgery.

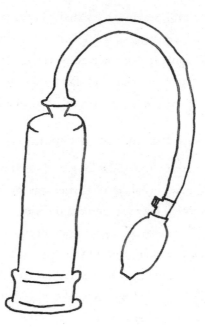

3) Penis pumps. You have probably seen these devices adver-
tised in the back of porn magazines. You insert your penis
inside a clear cylinder that is attached to an electric or
hand pump, which you squeeze manually. When pumped,
the cylinder will create suction that in effect causes your
blood vessels to become engorged. Your penis may feel
bigger. It may even look a bit bigger, but the moment you
remove the cylinder you begin to lose any effects. Pumps
are not great enlargement devices, but nonetheless many
men report enjoying the suction they cause.

4) Inflatable implants. Just like it sounds, a doctor can

implant cylinders into your shaft. These cylinders are connected to a pump that is implanted into your scrotum. You literally squeeze your balls to pump air into your penis. A release valve reverses the effect. This technique is used more for erectile dysfunction than size enhancement.

Can a penis be too long for a vagina?

Yes. He may have an especially long cock or she may have an especially short vaginal canal. If you have this problem I recommend experimenting with how you enter and thrust inside her. Her cervix is the back wall of her vagina, but it sticks out a little like the tip of your nose. Many women have a little extra space all the way around their cervix. If your penis and her vagina are compatible in shape, you may be able to find a direction of thrust that creates less impact directed on the tip of her cervix.

I also recommend experimenting with positions. You should be looking for positions that feel good but also create a shallower stroke. For example, she lies flat on her tummy with her partner entering her pussy from behind. If she is even a little voluptuous this position will make it so her thighs and butt keep your stroke shallow. With a slick lube however you will not feel like you are missing out on anything because her butt and thighs will envelop you. Hot!

Also note that she may be extra-sensitive to length a week or so before her period, when she is ovulating. At this point in her cycle her cervix drops down a little as a normal part of her cycle.

Do you have any tips if your partner is very large?

Vaginal tissue is built to be flexible (think childbirth). Use plenty of lube just to make it as easy as possible on your tissue. The hardest part of taking a larger penis is getting your vaginal or anal muscles to accept more size. For people with especially tight muscles this can be nearly impossible. Be patient with your body. Use any muscle-relaxing skills you may have. Do things like take a bath before you have sex or have him give you a nice body massage. When he is about to enter you be sure to take beep breaths. It should get easier with time. If not, change the focus of your sex play to less emphasis on penetration and more on hands, fingers, mouths, and sex toys.

Is a curved penis better than a straight one?

They certainly can be. A curved penis may look a little strange at first but they can be extremely effective in stimulating the g-spot or the prostate. The curve can also have an effect on the feeling of his thrust and how your muscles work around it.

But ultimately the only thing that matters is how skilled he is in using his penis and how well he understands how his partner gets off. If he understands what his goals are in pleasing his partner, he will be able to meet them. For example a female partner may respond to g-spot sensation, cervix bumping, fast strokes, slow stokes, or a male partner may respond to prostate stimulation or any variation of thrusting.

It's also up to you to look at your partner's shape and possible curve so you can figure how to get on that thing! Figure out where your g-spot or prostate is and point him in that direction.

Does having a pierced penis make sex better?

There are many individuals who find a penis piercing to be a very erotic, be it having themselves pierced or a lover who is pierced. For these people just having the piercing is enough to turn them on.

As for sex with a pierced penis, the response varies. I contacted Danica Gee, a professional body piercer who works at Tattoo Zoo in Victoria, British Columbia. She said, *"Everyone* will give you a different answer, but as I tell my clients: Piercing your penis may sound like it's going be a bonus for the other partner, but in reality it's usually just decorative. Women have the most sensation in the first two inches into the vagina. Those piercings at the head of their penis don't do much during sex other than tap around her cervix. All genital piercings I perform come with the disclaimer that they should be done with the idea that they are merely decorative, nonfunctional in a sexual way. If they do turn out to be sexually functional, then great, but I don't make any promises."

Danica also told me penis piercings can be painful during sex, as the in-and-out motion can pull on the piercings and cause some discomfort. Condoms and an abundance of lube tend to fix that.

9

Balls, Perineum, & Male Pelvic Muscles: Pleasure Beyond His Penis

I t is so easy to get sidetracked by his fabulous penis that you may totally overlook other erogenous areas on his body, like his balls! Sometimes called scrotum, these remarkable bits of anatomy can provide a wealth of pleasure.

In the womb, we all start out with the same basic genital form. Our pelvic skin can grow into labia lips or scrotum. If you are a female, use this fact as your guide for understanding how the skin on his balls may react to touch—very similar to your vaginal lips. Don't hesitate to explore this area of his body. Touch him the ways you like to have your lips touched, and see how he responds.

Just as a woman's body has its own unique shape, size, and response, the same is true for him. His balls appear big, full, small, deflated, short, long, any variation of color and any combination of these qualities.

FACT:

The average human testicle is 2 inches long and 1.2 inches in diameter. For most men the left side of his balls hangs lower than the right.

Does it feel good when you squeeze a guy's balls?

For some men it does. Other guys may like light strokes, hot breath, licks, light scratching, or nothing at all on their balls. You can determine how much pressure and sensation your guy likes by starting with a small amount of pressure and asking him, "Does this feel good?" Let him know you are trying to learn how to touch him. Ask him to show you how he likes it. Allow him to position your hand where he wants it and then use his hand over your hand to show you how he might do it.

" My current lover really enjoys it when I lick, tickle, and suck on his balls. He especially loves it when I get one in my mouth and press into his pelvis while humming. Straight out of the shower I can't get enough of licking and sucking and caressing his balls, perineum, and penis. Love it all. **"**

True Tales of Ball Pleasure:

"My balls are pretty sensitive, actually, and I can't have them scratched or tugged on too much. Having them held or gently jiggled is great, but anything more than that becomes a bit painful. I see a lot of porn videos where women suck on them, but that's not fun for me."

"I am amazingly amused by balls. The best part is blowing on them and watching the landscape shift like some alien planet. Plus they add to the joy of certain positions by slapping up against me. And they provide momentary distractions and opportunities for playfulness while giving oral sex. My last lover had incredibly sensitive balls, too, and his reactions got me even more involved."

"I love balls that are freshly shaven. They're really nice and soft and fun to play with. I don't like balls with hair all over them as it gets caught in my throat, and I don't like sweaty/sticky/smelly balls because, well, that's just not much fun."

"I think they are fairly unattractive. However, good sex involves as many parts as possible, so I'm always game to do whatever the guy likes to have done."

"I like to stroke or rub them while giving a blowjob or a hand job.

"I like balls. I like lightly scratching them with my nails and seeing what it makes my boyfriend do."

"I love my balls! My balls are big and bouncy! I love to have them held. Sometimes when we have sex, my wife will reach down and lightly scratch the back of my balls. It drives me wild. When I masturbate, I caress them and lightly scratch my fingernails along my sack."

"I dig the boyz, and I always feel as if they are chronically and systemically neglected and disenfranchised, and that it is up to me to make up years of being overlooked and slighted in favor of the penis. And a little trim goes a long way if you want them kissed or licked."

Stimulating his balls can be a great way to tune into his orgasmic response. When the two of you get comfortable with your hand on his balls, you will be able to feel his testicles draw up into his body a bit as he is about to orgasm. You become so tuned in with your partner that you start to recognize his very subtle responses to pleasure!

For some guys, when you feel his testicles draw up, you can very gently pull them down and postpone his orgasm. Controlling another person's orgasm like this can be a powerful way to play! But again, be gentle and stay tuned in with his response. Listen to his breath, watch how his body moves, and ask him yes-or-no questions so you can be sure you are driving his experience in the right direction.

What exactly is "blue balls" and do men really get this?

Blue balls is the slang term for *vasocongestion*, the temporary pain or discomfort some guys might feel when they have been sexually excited and do not reach orgasm. They may experience this when their blood vessels become engorged with blood and do not drain as fast as they would if they had ejaculated. This sensation can be subtle or more extreme, depending upon the guy.

One of the saddest things about vasocongestion is the misunderstanding of what it is and how to remedy the discomfort. Vasocongestion is not an illness or disease. In fact it is a normal bodily response.

Some men have been known to use this discomfort to manipulate their partner into bringing them to orgasm or following through with a sex act that the partner may not be prepared to do at that moment. Manipulation will never bring anything good into your sex play. If your body is really feeling pressure to get off, never use your situation to pressure your partner into getting you off. Keep in mind that this sensation does not last long and can be remedied by giving yourself an orgasm, taking a cool shower, or exercising.

Not only are his balls very sensitive and responsive to touch, they are also very pliable, giving you the opportunity to push them forward or back where you can reach more erectile tissue. If you use a couple of fingers you can massage the area where his balls meet his pelvic platform. Start at the top, penis side of his balls and you will feel his shaft extends deeper into his body and behind his balls. This is called the *root* of the penis and can extend two to three inches inside his body. He must have a full erection for you to feel his root.

Be gentle as you explore this area, and if you see he is responsive work your way up to more intense moves. Some men do not even know their shaft continues deeper into their body so this tissue may have never been touched or may be more sensitive simply because it does not get the same kind of play that the external shaft gets.

If you cup his balls in your hand and sort of bounce them,

pushing them up against his pelvic platform, you may find he loves
it. You are using his balls to stimulate erectile tissue that is directly
on the other side of his balls. Continuing back, past his balls you will
find the last bit of his root embedded in his perineum.

What is the perineum and where is it located?

The *perineum* is the area between his balls and his anus, and it is
another spot that can be an extremely responsive area for many men.
Not only does this spot allow you to access more erectile tissue from
the root of his penis, but just as with the female body all of the male
pelvic muscles come together at this one area.

FACT:

Though much of the ancient Chinese Taoist heritage has been
destroyed, we do know they had a very advanced sexual culture. They referred to the male perineum as "The Gateway to
Life and Death" because of the extreme sexual response one
may find there.

This is the spot where you should try using your fingers, tongue,
and/or vibrator on him. When using your fingers I recommend
using the pads of two or three of your fingers, rather than the pinpoint pressure of a single finger. Imagine this: you are face-to-face
with his balls in your hand. Your fingers inch back to his perineum.
Use your finger pads to create rhythmic pressure, pushing into his
body, or do a firm circular massage.

HOMEWORK:

There are so many guys who are shy about having their butt or anywhere near their anus touched. You know your guy is butt-shy if you try to reach any farther back than his balls and you see him jump or tense up his muscles. Sometime we think it's fun to tickle our partner or see him jump, but if you want to explore this area of his body you will have to teach him how to relax in your hands. Here's how:

1) In the normal course of using you hands on his shaft, slide your hand down onto his balls.
2) Before you get so far back that he will get tense, with your warm hand still on his balls, let him know your plans. Say to him, "I want to touch your perineum. I know you are ticklish around there, but I promise I won't touch your butt."
3) If he is agreeable, then slide your fingers back onto his perineum, using your finger pads to create a rhythmic pressure, or do a firm circular massage. Tune in and gauge his response.

But whatever you do, *don't touch his anus!* You are showing him he can trust you. Keep your promise. With a little time and practice he will be able to relax in your hands and experience new heights of pleasure with you, around his perineum and elsewhere perhaps! If all goes well and the two of you are turned on by these techniques, this could be the beginning of eroticizing his butt area and possibly opening up his mind to anal play.

Why do I get little response from my guy when I touch his perineum?

Just as with any other part of the body, it's important that you tune in to your partner's unique response to being touched in this area. He may love this sensation or he may hate it. He may want a very soft touch or he may want some extreme pressure. If he is not into it, no big deal. Just go to those hot spots that always deliver!

Is the perineum as pleasurable of a spot on a woman as it is on a man?

Guys tend to have the most extreme response to perineum stimulation. Women have some erectile tissue here and lots of muscles, but men have pelvic muscles, a direct connection to their shaft because the root is located here, and you can use the erectile tissue of his root to stimulate his prostate from the outside of his body. It only makes sense that his response would be more intense than her response. But again, every body is unique.

Where is the prostate located?

The *prostate* is inside his body, above the root of his penis and below his bladder. It is one of three glands that build seminal fluid. It goes like this; the semen is created in his testicles. When he is ready to come his balls draw up a little as they get ready to release semen into the sperm ducts. The ducts are just two tubes that bypass his bladder and connect directly into his urethra. But along the way they connect to three glands that add seminal fluid into the mix. The seminal fluid protects the sperm in cases where it may meet the alkaline fluids in a woman's vagina. The prostate is his biggest gland and builds the majority of his ejaculate fluid. It's a major player in his orgasm.

If you look at the illustration you can see that by pushing on his perineum you are using the root of his penis to put pressure on his prostate. If done at the right time this may cause some men to come instantly!

Where is a guy's g-spot?

Sometimes the people refer to the prostate as the "male g-spot" or the "p-spot." This is because the female g-spot and the prostate are both internal areas of the body that may induce orgasms for some people. In one scientific study of the fluid that the female g-spot (urethral sponge) creates, female "ejaculate" was compared to the prostate glandular fluid. In my opinion it is all a bit speculative, but that is why you may find reference to a male g-spot or p-spot.

One more important factor in the perineum are the *male pelvic muscles*. As with women's pelvic muscles, these are an important part of his overall health and orgasmic response as well. When he orgasms these muscle contract involuntarily: the stronger his pelvic muscles, the more control he will have over his orgasm and the stronger his orgasms can be.

Strong pelvic muscles have also been associated with a healthy prostate. These muscles surround the prostate gland and squeeze the prostate with orgasm and in the process help prevent swelling or hardening of the prostate.

Many men experience multiple orgasms by studying ancient sex practices that focus on breathing and pelvic muscles. These practices encompass exercises and mastering the art of becoming conscious in your body. I highly recommend men and lovers of men read *The Multi-Orgasmic Man*, by Mantak Chia and Douglas Abrams. This is the single greatest resource I have ever found on male anatomy and expanding male pleasure.

How to Exercise Male Pelvic Muscles

Locate your muscles. These are the same muscles you use when you are trying to stop the flow of pee. If it helps, just once stop the flow of pee. You will feel your pelvic muscles in your perineum rise up. I do not recommend stopping the flow of pee if you do not have to. This can cause reflux (urine going back up your urethra) and in some cases lead to urinary tract infections. But do it just once if you need to find these muscles.

Focus directly on the pelvic floor muscles, not your stomach muscles or you upper thigh and butt muscles.

As with any exercise, the more you do them the easier they get.

1) Get an erection.
2) Stand sideways in front of the mirror and bounce your erection up and down. Doing this move may look funny to you at first but it's really a fun and healthy thing to do.
3) Do twelve repetitions. And repeat.
4) Be sure to breathe.

If you are looking to kick it up a notch, take a wet washcloth and drape it over your erection. This way you are weight lifting with your cock.

Some guys also like to flex these muscles while in a relaxed state, or while having solo or partnered sex. Any flexing you can do just adds to your strength and ultimately to your orgasmic response!

10.

Butt: The Equal Opportunity Orifice

Everyone has the possibility of finding pleasure in their butt! Whether or not you want to go there (as a receiver or giver) is a personal choice. If for any reason you are one of the many butt-shy people in this world, please remember there is no harm in reading on and understanding your anal anatomy, because it is your butt and you should understand yours.

The *anus* is the external opening. It may be any skin color. The anus is usually darker that the rest of your butt because it is gathered skin that is loaded with blood vessels and nerve endings. Like much of our pleasure anatomy it may get darker when sexually excited.

The nerve endings in the anus are highly responsive. There is some erectile tissue in this area but the responses are heightened even more because everyone's butt has little hairs around the opening. They may be so light that you cannot see them or they may

FACT:

A recent anal bleaching fad has some people seeking to change the color of the skin around their anal opening, believing the more pink their anal opening is the cleaner it looks. Some waxing salons have begun to offer anal bleaching sessions where, for about seventy-five dollars, someone will wax your butt hairless and apply a cream that is similar to the creams that remove age spots and other skin discolorations. The truth is that the pigmentation around the anal sphincter is naturally darker for most people and determined by genetics. Just like some people are taller while others are short. Your butt hole may be browner while someone else's is pinker. I recommend you save your money and just declare your ass to be perfect as it is. Anyone who loves you will agree.

be dark and obvious. But these little hairs create response so you don't even have to touch the skin to get a reaction. You can even get a reaction from simply blowing air over your lover's anus. It's fun!

Some people like to have their anus massaged with a vibrator, a slippery finger, the pads of a few fingers, or the shaft of a penis. Your partner may want an external massage and nothing more. Or this can be a wonderful way to eroticize this area and warm them up for something more.

The anus and entire anal canal is made up of some extremely

delicate tissue. Part of the reason you will need to be more cautious is because the anal opening is not self-lubricating. Always use quality lube with anal play. The lube on a condom will not be enough lube for comfortable anal play. Also look carefully at any instruments you may insert in the butt. Make sure your toys are completely smooth and your fingernails are short and rounded.

How clean is the average person's butt hole?

To be honest I have never seen a study done on this subject. I am sure it depends upon the individual, their digestive health, and their personal hygiene habits. Even with the cleanest person there can be trace amounts of poop and bacteria. If you are concerned about cleanliness, foreplay in the shower is a great way to put your mind at rest. Shower or no shower, always be sure to use safer sex barriers with anal play. Condoms can cover your penis, toys, or fingers and a smooth, lubricated glove can be extremely exciting in anal play.

How dangerous is it to put your mouth on someone's anus?

This is called *rimming* or *analingus*. It's not very safe. As I said, even the cleanest person can have trace amounts of feces, which could expose you to hepatitis A, parasites and viruses, and in more rare cases HIV/AIDS.

You can safely go down on your partner's anus by using a safer sex barrier. You can use a dental dam, a condom that has been cut lengthwise, a piece of a latex glove, or even plastic wrap (like the kind you use in the kitchen to cover food). Put a little lube on your lover's anus to help hold your barrier in place and create a little wetness to go with the warmth of your mouth. They get that same amazing oral sensation

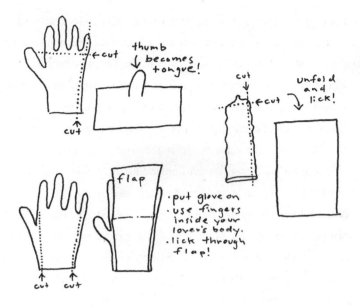

and you get the peace of mind of knowing your mouth is healthy. I recommend keeping a few of these barriers in your sex kit so they are ready to use and/or keeping a scissors in your kit so you can whip up a barrier to fit whatever sex play you may be having.

Why do people like anal sex?

For many people it feels good. For some people anal penetration, along with clitoral or penis stimulation, can help build more pressure in their pelvis and heighten their orgasmic response. Other people can orgasm from anal sex without added stimulation. Some women report feeling g-spot stimulation through anal sex because the walls that separate the anal and vaginal canals are rather thin, while men can easily achieve prostate stimulation through anal sex.

Beyond the physical stimulation, a lot of people enjoy the

psychological aspects of doing something that is considered to be taboo or naughty. For most people having anal sex requires a high level of trust and submission, which can be highly arousing.

There are also numerous situations where a person should not have anal sex. Don't have anal sex just to please your partner. I always say the number one thing you need in order to have great anal sex is desire. If you do not want to do it for your own sense of pleasure, then it will be hard to relax and enjoy it. Only have anal sex if you want to explore it for your own pleasure.

Don't have anal sex in order to experience intercourse without the fear of getting pregnant. Having anal sex instead of vaginal sex is not a reliable birth control method. Semen could still seep into your vagina during or after sex play. If this is you, I would recommend finding an alternative method of birth control, like condoms. Or consider other ways of having fun that do not require penetration.

Don't have anal sex if you think it means you will be able to maintain your status as a virgin. Some misguided young people have anal sex because they believe as long as they have no vaginal penetration they are still virgins. This can happen because the individuals involved have never had medically accurate, comprehensive sex education or because their culture requires that young women have an intact hymen in order to be eligible for marriage.

Can women orgasm from anal sex?

Yes. Both women and men can orgasm from anal sex. The sphincter muscles are part of the pelvic muscle group. With every orgasm there is what they call *anal response*. Anal responses are the involuntary contractions that happen in the sphincter muscles as the entire pelvic platform gets rocked by an orgasm. If you could see your butt while you were orgasming (don't ask me how!) you would see your anus sort of winking with every muscular contraction.

If you are a woman who is receiving anal sex, you can bring enough blood and oxygen into your pelvis to inspire an orgasm. Because your muscles trigger the orgasm (as opposed to a clit-triggered orgasm) it can be very intense. I have even met a number of women who can *only* orgasm through anal sex.

The strong ring of *sphincter muscles* creates the puckering of skin around the anus. The next time you are in the shower insert your own soapy finger into your butt. You will find it slips in rather easily and you can feel the grip of these muscles.

The ring of muscles is about one to two inches deep and made of two sets of muscles. The outer muscles we can control consciously. You know this muscle well. You can take a moment right now, close your eyes, take a deep breath, and relax your external sphincter muscles.

While doing this exercise you will notice that you did not poop yourself, right? That is because you have a second set of internal muscles that are controlled primarily by your autonomic nervous system. The same system that controls your breathing and heartbeat. You can, however, send cues to the inner muscles by relaxing your outer muscles because the two sets work in conjunction with each other as anal gatekeepers.

How much anal stimulation do men and/or women like?

That depends upon the person. Some people want light external stimulation only. Others want a slow in-and-out movement with a finger or a toy. Some people do not like an in-and-out movement but prefer the consistent pressure of a butt plug. The only way to know how much anal stimulation you or your partner may like would be to explore all your options and talk to each other about which types of stimulation feel best for you.

MYTH:

Many people have heard that having anal sex will stretch out your butt, cause damage, or even make it so that you have to wear a diaper the rest of your life. Fear not! Having anal sex in a healthy way can actually strengthen your anal muscles and be good for your butt because it encourages blood flow into your muscles.

The only time I have heard of people damaging their butt is if they have anal sex while being drunk or high on drugs. Drugs inhibit our ability to feel pain. Good anal sex should never be painful. If you feel pain it is an indication that you may need more lube, you may need to take a deep breath and relax your muscles, or you may need to stop. An impaired person does not get those signals and may end up getting hurt.

Beyond this two-inch ring of muscles is the *rectum*. The rectum is about five inches long. It is not a slick walled orifice like the vagina but instead the soft rectum walls sort of snake around toward the navel and then toward the spine to create an S shape. You need to enter a person's body slowly so you can accommodate the unique curves of their rectum.

Most people find the bulk of their pleasure in the muscles of their anal canal, while others like the fullness that comes with having something larger filling their rectum. The only way to know how you or your lover will respond to these kinds of stimulation is to experiment and talk to each other about what you are feeling.

Men can have a response to anal penetration that is unique to them because they have a *prostate*. The prostate is about two inches inside, toward the naval. You can stimulate it by inserting your finger and doing a gentle "come here" motion toward his navel. His prostate may feel a bit firmer as he gets closer to ejaculating. For some men even a slight amount of pressure on their prostate will inspire an orgasm. Other guys need the massaging action that comes from toys or a penis. This is one of those sensations that a man has a difficult time performing on himself.

At the end of the rectum there is another sphincter called the *rectosigmoid sphincter*. This is a very important bit of our anatomy that helps a lot of people feel more at ease with anal penetration. It is another circular band of muscles that separates the rectum from the *colon*. Poop is stored in the colon. When a person is ready to poop, the rectosigmoid sphincter opens and lets the poop down into the rectum. We can feel this happening. Think about the signals your body gives you when you have to poop. You feel a specific nudge in your bowels. I call it the "Ten-Minute-Warning Bell." For some people it could be a thirty-minute bell or a two-minute bell. Most of the time there is no poop in your rectum because your rectum is merely a passageway.

If you are not pooping normally on a given day, then avoid anal sex and just concentrate on letting your butt be healthy. Those individuals who have chronic pooping problems like constipation or diarrhea usually have an over- or underactive rectosigmoid sphincter. If you have chronic pooping problems, anal sex may not be the best kind of sex for you.

If we are having anal sex will he actually be touching poop inside my body?

If he wants to have anal sex with you he should wear a condom and be adult enough to understand your butt's primary function. There may be some residue because poop does exit through your rectum. So, yes, occasionally there will be a little poop residue on him. The rectum is not a storage space for poop. It is a passageway. If you have had a regular, healthy poop that day, there should be no poop in your rectum.

If you feel hesitant to go there because you are afraid you will be embarrassed by poop, you may want to give him this little disclaimer, "You know what my butt is used for. If there is any poop, it's on you!" Then you have cleared the air, voiced your concerns, and given him the option to not go there if he is worried about poop.

Is there any way to sort of rinse out my butt before anal sex?

You can give yourself an enema or anal douche. An enema is a bottle or bag with a nozzle that is used to inject warm water into the rectum. An anal douche is a smaller bottle with less liquid that can be used to do a quick rinse of the rectum. But if you have had a healthy poop that day and have had a shower recently, this is not necessary. If you still prefer rinsing out your body, you can buy an enema at any pharmacy. Empty out the liquid in the bottle because it is a diuretic and will inspire loose stools. (Not sexy!) Fill it up with lukewarm water and follow the directions on the box. Or there is an item called an anal douche that you can buy at most sex shops.

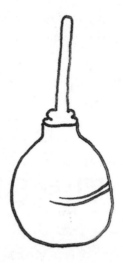

Are you not supposed to mix vaginal and anal body fluids?

True! You can go from vaginal play to anal play but never put anything that has been used in anal play into the vagina. The butt has all sorts of bacteria that help keep it healthy and fight infection. But these bacteria can actually inspire infections in the urethra or vagina. It's the same reason why women are taught to wipe from front to back. I also recommend using a thicker lube for anal play so that any lube you apply to the anal region stays in the anal region and does not run into her vagina.

In the end, it's your anatomy and it's yours to explore. Some feel more comfortable exploring during solo play, while others would rather hand themselves over to their lover like a hot science experiment. Understanding where your hot spots may be is the first step in understanding how to go about exploring them. Enjoy!

11.

Body Image:
The Skin You're In

I am sexy. I am flawed. I have blemishes, scars, stretch marks, body hair, and a big butt. But I am very sexy. Why? I gave up on trying to meet unrealistic standards. I decided to be as kind to myself as I am to others. I accept myself as I am and look to find healthy ways to be the best I can be.

People who accept and love themselves are powerful people and usually people who do well in all aspects of their lives, including sex. It was Roseanne Barr who said, "The thing women have got to learn is that nobody gives you power. You just take it." Look in the mirror and take back your power. Accept the fact that you—like everyone—are flawed. Accept the fact that your body never stops growing and changing. This is a normal, healthy fact of life.

I struggled through puberty as a flat-chested tomboy, and then grew breasts that were so big my own sister looked at me one day and asked if I had secretly gotten implants. I'm in my midthirties now and notice my hips are a bit wider. My weight goes up and down. Over the years I have looked at my body and wondered if I was pretty. Is my butt *too* big? Does my vagina taste right? Should I shave my pubes into a racing stripe or should I do that Brazilian wax thing I hear people talking about? I have compared my body to those of friends, magazine models, and porn stars. It seems the questions are endless and they change with each passing year.

Society (with the help of Photoshop) keeps perpetuating ideas that are unrealistic. Women should be perfectly hairless. Skin is flawless and glistening. Men don't cry. Pussy smells like fish. Fat people are funny. Men who are well groomed are gay. Disabled people do not have sex. It's all lies.

Like most of us I work hard to overcome self-doubt and find peace in my body. I have learned to live without shame, to have no regrets, and to live life to the fullest no matter what anyone thinks of my decisions. I pull these body image questions apart, speak with other women, read every empowering book I can get my mittens on. And I am still learning how to accept myself just as I am and how literally to have sex with the lights on.

How can I project sexiness if I am not happy with my body?

Sexiness has very little to do with your body. A sexy person can be of any size, age, color, religion, or ability. I ask a few friends which well-known people, who defy typical media-induced ideas of sexy, do they find to be oh-so-sexy? They told me, Queen Latifah for her size-defying beauty. Funny, sexy geeks like Jon Stewart, Janeane Garofalo, and Conan O'Brien. The ever changing Madonna and David Bowie. And, of course, there is Susan Sarandon—who only gets hotter with age!

Sexy is in your spirit and mind. You exude it through your body language, verbal language, hygiene, and self-respect. I promise you— your body is secondary to all of those things.

I asked more than five hundred people what makes a person sexy. Here are their top answers:

1. Smiling
2. Confidence
3. Sense of humor
4. Attitude
5. Playfulness
6. Eyes
7. Intelligence
8. Imagination/creativity
9. Being uninhibited
10. Being adventurous
11. Style
12. Flirtatiousness
13. Communication
14. Independence

If you look at this list you will notice that the top answers were not "big boobs," "small boobs," "tummy," "flat tummy," "big butt," or "thin thighs." Instead you have an entire list of things that are totally attainable by anyone.

Want to be sexier? Smile. Laugh. Forgive your flaws because we all have them. Put your chin up. Sing. Dance. Look your lover in the eyes. Read. Learn. Try new things. Flaunt. Flirt. Dress up. Ask for what you want. Listen to you lover. Indulge in the things that make you happy.

HOMEWORK:

Get a blank sheet of paper and write the numbers one to fourteen down one side. Go through the list above of what makes a person sexy and write down one action you can take to bring more of that quality into your life. This sheet of paper will be your to-do list. And you will become even sexier.

I'm a handsome guy that just happens to be handicapped and in a wheelchair. I've tried using the online dating stuff and the girls seem interested until they find out I'm in a wheelchair, then they stop talking. Any advice on how I could get and keep them interested?

Your mission: Don't give up! Keep putting yourself out there and meeting more women. If someone rejects you because of your wheels, they are shallow. Move on to the next conquest. You need to be persistent and continue to be your charming self.

Try flirting with women in more face-to-face situations, like at the library, on the street, and in the grocery store. If you see someone who sparks your interest, go for it! The worst-case scenario is that they say no. The best-case scenario is that you find someone who sees past your disability and into your handsome, lustful heart!

A possible online option is a www.dateable.org. DateAble is a unique nonprofit social organization for people with and without disabilities who seek new friends and relationships.

Also check out the Resources section at the back of this book. *The Ultimate Guide to Sex and Disability* is chock-full of amazing material including lots of first-person advice from super-sexy disabled individuals. They deliver information on how to have great sex and how to speak with partners about your body and desires. Another one of my favorite books, *Guide to Getting It On!,* is full of great information and very inclusive when it comes to disabilities. I hope you will pick up these books and let them inspire you!

FACT:

Great sex happens when you find a position that is comfortable for your body. This can be especially difficult if you are disabled, pregnant, or suffering from an injury. However ablebodied you may be, I suggest checking out the Liberator sex ramps and cushions (theliberator.com) and the Body Bouncer (bodybouncer.com). Unique sex accoutrements like these take the pressure off your body and bring more pleasure into your sex play.

How can I get rid of stretch marks?

Stretch marks are normal. They are the result of damage that has been done to the deep fibers of your skin. Stretch marks can happen to people in puberty if they have a rapid growth spurt, individuals who gain fat or muscle at a rate or scale that their skin cannot adapt to, and to most women who have babies. They start out as red marks that fade with time and become less noticeable. These scars are difficult and sometimes impossible to repair.

You can make an appointment with a dermatologist and have them assess your stretch marks to see if there are any possible treatment options for you. Sometimes they use a cream called Retin-A (not recommended for nursing moms) or do laser treatment. If you are pregnant or have fresh stretch marks you may want to try using vitamin E oil or cocoa butter creams to limit the stretch marks that may occur or help heal new stretch marks.

Your best option may be to forgive your stretch marks and look at them as a map of where you have been. A story on your skin of weight loss, muscle strength, babies being born.

One day I was reading an article about sexy siren Salma Hayek (a body image heroine of mine!). She was talking about the stretch marks on her body and referred to them as "tiger stripes." Meow! Suddenly I felt a whole lot better about my stripes, too.

How do I get over my hang-ups about my big thighs?

Feeling bad about your thighs (or any other part of your body) is not going to solve the issue. You really only have two choices—change your thighs or learn to love them. If you can make your thighs slimmer and do it in a healthy way (that is, without surgery or excessive dieting or exercise), do it.

If for some reason you cannot change your thighs, then please take a deep breath, forgive your flaws, and go back and look at your three best physical features. Those are the things that your lover will zero in on. A person who is attracted to you will always concentrate on what they love the most about your body. That is the magic of love, lust, and attraction!

Every Naked Moment

We used to have a light switch in the bathroom that would dim the lights with a twist of the wrist. I was very fond of that feature and would take advantage of it when my boyfriend (now husband) would invite me into the shower. I would dim the lights and say, "How about a little romance?" And I would giggle with the anticipation of what was to come.

I never thought much about it until one evening when he actually answered my rhetorical question, "Can we leave the lights on for once? I just want to see you."

What? I was a little caught off guard. He had never said that before and suddenly I was struck with the reality of what I was doing. I was using the dimmer to hide. Hide my body.

I am a sex educator. Shouldn't I have the power to be naked? People always imagine me having the best sex ever—swinging from the chandeliers, living every fantasy, and being a free spirit. And here I was, unable to be naked. Shit.

I told him the truth. "I have these scars on my tummy. I hate them. I don't want you to look at them," I said, gesturing toward the area under my navel where I had multiple surgeries as a child to repair birth defects.

"I don't care about those scars. You can barely see them. I just want to look at your boobs! You have the best tits ever. . . ." And then he lost himself in this ridiculous rant about my boobs that was far too funny and long to remember. He loves my boobs.

Later that evening while lying in bed a revelation hit me. Here I was spending every naked moment concentrating on the part of my body that I hate the most, desperately and discreetly trying to find creative ways to cover my scars and hide my body. All the while he was spending every one of my naked moments concentrating on the part of my body he loves the most.

I was being so hard on myself. I would not treat my best friend or my boyfriend in this manner. Why would I do this to myself? I vowed that I would be nicer to myself. I would try to see my body through his eyes. I would not let these scars ruin my naked moments.

These days I am more kind to myself. I don't bother trying to cover my scars or hold my stomach in. I let my mascara run and my hair is a wild mess. We have more uninhibited sex. Great sex! It's not always easy but I try to follow my husband's lead and do my damnedest to spend my every naked moment concentrating on the parts of my body I love the most.

What are some of the ways you were able to overcome feeling shame?

Shame is not a progressive emotion. It does not bring anything good into your life. People will attempt to cast shame on others as a means to control, manipulate, and belittle them. Beware of anyone who attempts to shame you. If you do experience shame it should be a fleeting emotion that catapults you into action.

For example, let's say you are ashamed of something you did once, like maybe you had unsafe sex one day last week. Take action. Make a doctor's appointment to get tested for any sexually transmitted diseases. Buy safe sex supplies and store them in your backpack, purse, glove box, or bedside so you will have them the next time you are intimate with someone. Tell your lover you have decided you feel bad when you take risks like having unsafe sex, so from now you are using condoms every time you have sex. Forgive yourself and do better next time.

I think my pussy smells bad. What should a woman's body smell like?

You could smell tangy, musky, or like sweat. Each woman will have her own unique scent. How good or bad your scent is really is in the nose of the beholder! You may think you smell bad but your lover may think you have the most delicious pussy ever. It's all relative to the individual.

If your pussy starts to smell funny or if you have unusual discharge, it could be a sign that your vaginal ecology is off kilter and that you need to see a doctor. You could have a yeast infection, bacterial infection, or sexually transmitted disease. The best thing you can do is see a doctor right away and take good care of yourself.

How to Keep Your Pussy Healthy

The vagina is amazing. It has its own carefully balanced ecology and when it's in working order, it's totally self-cleaning.

All a woman needs is to shower with water to stay fresh and clean. But there are so many things we do to our bodies that can throw off our natural ecology. Here are some tips to help keep your pussy healthy!

1) Don't douche. If you are having issues with your vaginal scent, douching will only aggravate the problem. Douching may rinse away bad bacteria, but it also rinses away the good bacteria. The good bacteria in your vagina is there to fight off foreign bacteria and infections. The best thing you can do is wash your vagina with water. If the problem persists see your gynecologist.

2) Avoid products with fragrance, like soaps, feminine sprays, powders, wipes, tampons, pads, and toilet paper. They only temporarily mask odor and can be irritating for many women. I know they market these products as if they are a great way to stay clean, but remember their real mission is to sell the product. Your health is not first on a big corporation's list of priorities.

3) Learn your scent. How do you smell? Have you ever tasted your own vagina? You should! A healthy vagina smells good, especially to our lover(s). The number one reason why men steal women's panties (and they do!) is because they love our scent. Not only that, you can use your scent to monitor your vaginal health. If you smell funny or you feel burning or itching, see a doctor.

4) Spermicide can irritate. A large percentage of women are allergic to the spermicide Nonoxynol-9. It is used on a lot of condoms, in birth control sponges, and diaphragm gels. If you or your partner experience inflammation after sex, or symptoms that you associate with yeast infections, you may want to seek out safer sex and birth control products without Nonoxynol-9.

5) Vaginal allergies are not uncommon. Some women experience allergies when they use lubricants. There are lots of lubes on the market, and picking the one for you is not that different from choosing the right hand lotion or eyedrops for your body. If you try one and it does not work, try a different one. Many shops have little sampler tubes of lubes, and that may be an easier way to find the right one for you. You may have adverse reactions to ingredients like glycerin, alcohol, flavors, or menthol. Read the ingredients list and be an informed consumer.

6) Beware of sugar during sex play. Whipped cream, chocolate syrup, and other sugary product can be fun when slathered on your body for your lover's tongue, but if they get in your vagina they can throw off your natural balance. If you are going to use sweet products, use them everywhere, but not in your vagina. You can even use them on your clit, but be conscious to not get them inside your body.

7) Use your mouth. If you think something (lube, condom, or toy) might be irritating your vagina, taste it. The membranes in your mouth are a lot like the membranes in your vagina, except you have the benefit of having taste buds. If the item or product tastes bad or numbs your mouth, you will probably want to avoid putting it in your vagina.

Do you recommend shaving or waxing?

I have tried both and think they are both great options if you are looking to groom your pubic hair. There is of course no reason that you have to shave or wax. Some people do it because they like the feeling of exposed skin, some do it because their lover can deliver better oral sex without the hair getting in the way, some do it because they like the way it looks, and others do it to turn on their lover.

Shaving is a simple way to freshen up your look and feel. But after a day or so it can leave you with razor burn, stubble, or bumps from ingrown hairs. Using a new multiblade razor and quality shaving cream will give you the best shave. In the shaving section of any big pharmacy you will find a plethora of products on the market that can help you combat all of those problems.

One thing I like about shaving is that you can get very creative with it. You can do the swimsuit triangle, the racer stripe, a postage stamp or even a heart on Valentine's Day!

Waxing can be more intense. Usually it means going to a salon and having a professional do it for you. It can be painful the first couple of times they do it but gets easier with each session. Waxing will leave most people free of hair for a few weeks. For many people hair grows back feeling softer because the entire hair is pulled out, root and all. There are no blunt edges like you have when hair is shaved.

—— · —— · ——

True Tales of Shaving (Or Not):

"I shave every morning in the shower. It really doesn't take long after you get used to doing it. Plus, it makes my cock look a little bigger!"

"I like a shaved partner because I don't like getting hair in my mouth when I go down on her."

"I'm middle-of-the-road. I don't like being completely shaven, nor do I like unkempt pubic hair. I keep mine trimmed."

"It's a hassle sometimes but I'm a shaver. I like the smoothness and somehow I also feel cleaner that way."

"I like pubic hair. I feel creepily prepubescent when clean shaven. A nice set of pubic curls is particularly erotic for me."

"I don't shave anything myself—I just hate shaving. On others I don't mind hair. I like to pet it when we're just cuddling. Shaven though is also nice—soft and smooth. The con for that comes when it's stubbly—stubble burn!"

"I only shave when I have a hot date, and I always leave a fairly largish triangle on top. I don't like the completely bald look and for some reason, that area also is the most irritating when it grows back."

❝ I love to shave because all the sensations seem heightened. And I far prefer a lover to be trimmed or shaved, especially if I'm going down on them. But I can deal with it if they're hairy. **❞**

How can I get my girlfriend to shave or wax?

It's her body. Ultimately she may turn you down, but the best advice I can give you is to tell her you believe her shaved pussy is beautiful. Don't tell her she's hot or that it gets you hot, the word here is *beautiful.* Women want and need to feel beautiful. Tell her you love her pussy, how it looks and smells. And that you would just once love to see it bare. If you get her to do it once, make sure you remind her how much you love the sight and feel of her shaved skin.

You should also offer to shave your own pubic area at the same time. This may help her feel more at ease with the idea. Plus, this way you'll have a lot more sympathy when she complains about shaving bumps!

HOMEWORK:

Has anyone ever given you an explicit sexual compliment on your body? When someone gives you a compliment on your sexual anatomy it makes you want to strip off your clothes and do something juicy! Think about your lover's body and give them one honest compliment. (I say *honest* compliment because you cannot tell your lover he has the *biggest penis you have ever seen.* Unless of course it is!) Tell her she has a beautiful pussy. Let him know you love the curve of his cock. Confess your adoration for her breasts. Hold his balls in your hand and tell him you like how firm they are. It's a great way to amp up your sex life and brings more positive energy into your sex play!

12

Sexual Health: Self-Care & Medical Care

How many times a week should a couple have sex in a normal, healthy sex life?

There is no such thing as normal. What is far more important than any statistic is thinking about what makes you and your lover happy. Perhaps the two of you like to have sex three times a day. If both of you are happy with that, then that is normal for you. Or maybe the two of you like to have sex once a month. If you are both happy with that, then that is also normal.

Never compare yourself to statistics, magazine articles, or stories you hear from friends. It's an unfair thing to do to you. Instead, talk to your lover and find the medium ground between the two of you. Check in periodically to see if you are both happy. If you feel like you want more or less sex play in your life, tell your partner. Ask them how they feel as well.

More important than frequency is creativity. Find ways to shake it up every now and then with some spontaneous sex. Use a highlighter pen on this book and highlight anything that sparks for you. Then pass the book to your lover. Give them a highlighter pen of another color and see what new things they may be interested in! If you get through the book, move on to exploring sex toys, games, more books, and erotica.

With that said, studies show the average number is 2.5 times a week. But who cares?

How can I boost my sex drive?

The number one cause for lowered libido is fatigue. When you add up the factors in your life you'll find you are juggling any combination of work, school, relationships, kids, social obligations, illness, or who knows what! Life's demands can be overwhelming. One of the best things you can do for your sex life and for your life as a whole is slow down.

Redefine what is important to you. Learn when to say no to people and events that are lower on your priority list.

Find healthy ways to care for yourself. Go for a walk, with your partner or alone. Cook and eat together. Exercise. Budget your money better so you can work less. Get a baby-sitter. Play board games. Stargaze. Relax. None of these things sound particularly sexy but these subtle changes will reconnect you with yourself, your lover, and your true priorities.

Beyond fatigue, our emotions have an impact on our sex life. You may need to assess your mental health and look at the amount of anxiety, shame, anger, and depression you carry. These emotions can cripple your sex drive. You can work through these problems by talking with friends and lovers, finding a mental health professional, seeking out group therapy, reading self-help books, and making a journal to sort your thoughts.

Antidepressants killed my sex drive. What can I do?

Talk to your doctor. There are so many medications on the market today that are helping people fight depression, so you should be able to find an alternative or possibly change the dosage of the one you are taking. This is true for other pharmaceuticals as well, like birth control pills. With the help of your doctor you will need to do some experimenting to find the right balance for your body. The only person who can help make this happen for you is your doctor.

How to Find a Sex-Positive Doctor

Having a healthy sex life is an important part of a person's overall health. Whether you are looking for a good general practitioner, gynecologist, or other specialists it's always good to know you can ask your health professional honest questions about things that affect your sexuality.

The first thing you need to know is that doctors receive a limited amount (if any) training in sexuality. Consequently many doctors bring their personal morality and baggage into their office when it comes to sex. Some doctors refuse to "go there" and don't recognize sexuality as an important part of our personal health and the health of our relationships. While other doctors make it a point to study sexuality by reading all of the latest articles and subscribing to medical journals that address sex and health. It's up to you to sift through and find the doctors who recognize the correlations between health and sex. Here is how you can do that.

Start by asking your friends or a family member you trust. A personal recommendation is always a great first-level screening.

Get out your phone book or HMO/insurance listing and highlight the doctors that are available to you. If you are a female, you may want to request a female doctor, as they will always have a more intimate understanding when it comes to female anatomy and experiences like birthing a child and being a mother. If you are lesbian, gay, bisexual, or transgendered (LGBT) you may want to seek out a doctor or clinic that openly caters to marginalized individuals. LGBT clinics often employ doctors who are sexually sophisticated and open to individuals who live alternative lifestyles like sex workers, people who practice alternative sex practices like bondage or polyamory, people who have lots of tattoos or body piercings, and so on.

Call every listing that may possibly suit your needs and ask to speak to the doctor you will be seeing on the phone before you set your appointment. Any good office will take your number and have the doctor call you. If they refuse to let you speak with your potential doctor over the phone, chances are they will not have a lot of time for you during an office visit, either.

When the doctor does call, ask straight away, "I'd like to speak with you honestly about issues that might possibly be health related and that are affecting my sexuality. Is that something you are willing to address with me?"

Then listen to the response from the doctor and use your instincts to decide if you would like to make an appointment with her or him.

Once you have found a doctor who may meet your needs, it's time for you to be a good patient. Before your appointment, sit down and write out a list of all of your questions and bring that list with you to your appointment. This way if your time with your doctor is rushed you can make sure to ask your doctor each and every question on your mind.

I am a person who experienced some very extreme medical situations as a young child. Before I hop up on a gynecologist's table or have blood taken I will give the practitioner a little disclaimer like, "I have experienced some trauma in the past so this is not easy for me." Although it's not easy to admit that to a stranger, I find it really helps to soften the practitioner's edge and I get better care. If you have suffered sexual or medical trauma, let them know in advance. This gives your doctor a chance to understand your situation and deliver better care. My gynecologist now knows me well enough to move right through the procedure. She knows the longer it takes to complete a procedure, the more upset I get.

It's sometimes hard for an individual to remember that each of us is the ultimate authority of her or his own body. You are also the person paying that doctor for their services. You have the right to ask for what you need without shame. It takes courage to take these steps, but I promise doing this will bring you better medical care and you will be more likely to get your questions about your body and sexuality answered in a respectable manner. You deserve that.

As you look for a sex-positive doctor, it's also important to remember that doctors are human and they are not perfect. They are often overworked and spend every day listening to people's problems and complaints. It's a hard job. But there are good doctors out there who want to help you. You just need to do a little work to find them.

Does your sex drive change during your period?

Yes. Menstruation is one of the most obvious life cycles that affect libido. About a week or so before a woman's period she may feel especially sexually driven. It is during this time that a premenopausal woman is ovulating and her body is the most receptive to pregnancy. This is not true for all women, but most report they have waves of excitement that run in a monthly cycle. For some it can be the week during or after her period.

HOMEWORK:

If you are a woman I recommend writing your patterns down on a calendar and getting to know your cycles. Record rhythms in your body like desire, cramps, PMS, breast tenderness, food cravings, creativeness, high energy, low energy, lightness or heaviness of your flow, or any other waves you may feel. This can help you learn to forecast your cycles and learn to love it. Schedule events during your high-energy times and curl up on the couch to watch movies during your low-energy times. Plan a sexy weekend during your high high-desire times and bake cookies when you know you'll be craving them. Learn to work with your body rather than resent your body when it does not seem to be working with your scheduled plans, because your body is going to work this cycle whether you decide to accept it or not. You might as well learn to make the most of it!

Do those aphrodisiac creams made for women really work?

I do not use any of the excitement products on the market but I have heard some good reports and some not-so-good reports about clitoral gels and warming lubes. People seem either to love them or hate them. Your response will be determined by how your body reacts to the ingredients.

The most active ingredient in these products is menthol. If you were curious to try these creams you might take the smallest amount of menthol (for example you could use the tiniest amount of toothpaste or mouthwash with a menthol base) and try it on your nipples, penis head, or clit. I do not recommend using these inside your body. If the tingling sensation feels good, then explore some other products. If not, then you'll know to avoid excitement products.

To be honest I have a limited amount of faith in the multitude of goos and creams that are on the market. The companies that make these products are unregulated, which means they can freely make claims that have not necessarily been proven in trail case studies. Be a responsible consumer. Read ingredients lists and try to understand what you may be using on your body. Listen to your body and make smart choices for you.

How can you have an orgasm when you are drunk?

Drinking can help a lot of people lower their inhibitions and relax, in turn raising one's desire to have sex. One of the downsides to drinking is that it affects the central nervous system (brain and spinal cord), which controls virtually all body function. The alcohol blocks messages that are trying to get to the brain, including perception, emotion, movement, vision, and hearing. The more you drink, the less control you have over your system, including your sexual function. Sometimes the affects of alcohol will inhibit your ability to orgasm. For some this can happen with relatively little alcohol. The best way to heighten your ability to orgasm? Drink less or don't drink at all.

Why do I need to be drunk in order to have sex?

Sex can be intimidating. Sexual situations can make you feel self-conscious and vulnerable, and drinking can alleviate those feelings. Liquor can give a person courage, lower inhibitions, and make it easier to meet people. With all that said, the truth is that you do not *need* to be drunk to have sex—you choose to be drunk.

If you are accustomed to being drunk before you are intimate, learning to be intimate without liquor can be quite challenging, but certainly not impossible. If you use or have a history of using alcohol to lower your inhibitions I highly recommend reading *Awakening Your Sexuality*, by Stephanie S. Covington. If you are a person who has experienced sexual trauma I recommend reading *The Survivor's Guide to Sex*, by Staci Haines. Once you have developed an ability to have sex sober you will find it is a ton of fun! Your orgasms are heightened, your ability to communicate is strong, you are able to advocate for your needs (like insisting on safer sex), you can remember what you did, and you smell better!

If you do enjoy mixing your vices please remember that when you are drunk, your guard is down, and sometimes people are not as responsible as they could be. Be prepared. If you know you are going out and drinking, keep condoms, lube, and other safer sex supplies in your backpack, purse, or glove box. Studies show that the more a person drinks, the more sex partners they have—and, their behavior tends to be more risky. So, have fun, but be smart.

HOMEWORK:

One study reported 18 percent of adolescents were drinking at the time of their first intercourse. It's a sad fact that people start experimenting with sex at the same age that many also start experimenting with alcohol and drugs. Do your kids a favor and speak openly and honestly about the problems that one may encounter when mixing substances and sex.

What is the best condom for both men and women's pleasure?

There are so many great condoms on the market today! It is impossible for me to pick just one because they each have unique features. Here is a list of some of my favorites.

Crown.
A very affordable condom. I love them because they are high quality and reliable yet men say they feel more sensation through them than your average condom. Because they are inexpensive they are ideal for slapping over sex toys to ensure they are clean and free of bacteria.

Inspiral.
One of the most unique designs on the market, this condom has a flared tip with an ice-cream-cone twist in

the design. The flared tip allows more room for blood circulation at the head of his penis and the twisted design creates a subtle tug with each stroke. Guys love it.

Kimono Microthin.

A high-quality condom that used to be hard to find but now it's popping up in more convenience stores and pharmacies around the country. Now available in a larger size.

Mamba.

Smaller than your average condom. Perfect for those who need a snug fit.

Avanti.

This polyurethane condom is a great alternative for those who are allergic to latex. More expensive than a latex condom but a lot less expensive than a sexually transmitted disease or a pregnancy!

Lifestyles Kiss of Mint.

A nonlubricated condom that tastes like minty fresh toothpaste! It was designed specifically for oral sex. So suit up with something delicious and be safe!

These condoms are available at all high-quality sex shops. (See the Resources section at the back of this book to find a shop near you or online retailer.) I recommend buying sample packs of individual condoms and creating your own top condoms list!

— · — · —

How to Put a Condom on With Your Mouth

1) Make sure you are using a quality product. Check the

expiration date. If you open it and it feels sticky or dried out, throw it away and get another. Latex goes bad with age, so if it looks or feels odd, it is probably old or damaged. Don't use it!

2) Put the condom on after he has an erection. Be sure you are using a condom that fits. If it is too tight it may burst and/or restrict his circulation.

3) Put a drop or two of latex-safe lubricant inside the tip of the condom. Lubricant on the outside and the inside will help prevent tears and rips.

4) Squeeze the tip of the condom to leave some extra space. This is called the reservoir tip and it is necessary to catch all the cum. If you can't wait to get the condom on, and he's not completely erect, leave a little more space in the tip to make way for his full erection.

5) Pinch that tip between your front teeth and your tongue. So the brim of the condom is outside of your mouth.

6) Go down on his penis like you would if you were giving him a blowjob and use your lips to push the condom brim over the head of his penis.

7) You can use your lips or your hands to roll it down the shaft. For me, my mouth is not deep enough to get the condom all the way down to the bottom of his shaft, so I will go as far as I can and use my hand.

8) Practice makes perfect!

I know I'm always supposed to use condoms but I think they're giving me an infection. Am I crazy?

Nope. I've had similar problems myself. I have learned that I am allergic to Nonoxynol-9. It's a spermicide that was once believed to offer some protection against HIV and other sexually transmitted diseases. Lots of women are having reactions to Nonoxynol-9. You will find it in many brands of condoms, contraceptive sponges, and some lubricants.

Much of the medical community has not yet recognized the allergy issue that many women have with Nonoxynol-9. My gynecologist was no help with this issue. She kept giving me yeast infection medicine or saying there was nothing wrong with me. Finally I bought a ton of different kinds of condoms (lubed, nonlubed, latex, nonlatex, with Nonoxynol-9, without Nonoxynol-9) and just screwed my way through some trial-and-error tests until I found a condom that works for me.

A few of the products women may experience inflammation from include latex, glycerin (found in many lubricants), perfumes, deodorants, alcohol, lotions, and oils. These products can throw off vaginal pH and kill off the good bacteria that keep our vaginas healthy. A woman may have similar problems if she has obsessive hygiene habits or douches.

You need to experiment to find the products that work for you. And if after sex you have symptoms that resemble those of yeast infections or urinary tract infections, you should definitely see your doctor right away. I recommend writing down your symptoms and your habits in regard to sex on a calendar so that you can help your doctor pinpoint just what the trouble is.

How safe are condoms for preventing HIV infection?

According to Planned Parenthood, "condoms offer good protection against infection with HIV." The only sure way to prevent yourself from coming in contact with HIV is by not having sex, but abstaining from sex is not realistic for most adults.

You can get HIV by having anal, vaginal or, less commonly, oral sex. Protect yourself by having dry sex through your clothes, watching each other masturbate, kissing, cuddling, using toys (but not sharing them), or by having phone and computer sex play. If you are engaging in penetrative play, use a condom.

Other factors that could put you at risk for HIV include sharing contaminated needles, getting accidentally pricked with a contaminated needle, contaminated blood transfusions, childbirth, and breast-feeding.

FACT:

Lambskin condoms are a valid form of birth control but will not protect you from sexually transmitted infections. Unlike latex condoms, lambskin condoms are porous and may permit passage of viruses like HIV and other sexually transmitted diseases. Some people choose to use lambskin if they are sensitive to latex. Polyurethane condoms are an alternative method of STD protection for those who are latex-sensitive.

What are the statistics on lesbian transmissions of HIV?

Women can pass HIV and other sexually transmitted diseases. You specifically asked for statistics, but the Centers for Disease Control (CDC) does not keep a statistic on how many lesbians and bisexual

women have HIV. But according to LesbianSTD.com, a website
that is produced with the oversight of Dr. Jeanne Marrazzo of the
University of Washington, there are documented cases of women-
to-women HIV infections.

Transmission most likely occurs during menstruation, when a
woman already has an infection like vaginitis, or if the partners are
engaging in rough sex play that may break delicate vaginal membranes. The best way to protect yourself is to minimize your possible
exposure to blood, including menstrual blood. Avoid sex play that
may cause cuts, scratches, or abrasions and have safer sex supplies
available so when things get hot and heavy you are ready!

What is a dental dam?

A dental dam is a square sheet of latex designed to use as a barrier
between the mouth and genitals during oral sex. The best brand I
have found is the Glyde Dam. They even come in a variety of mild
flavors like vanilla and grape.

You put a little lube on her pussy and/or anus to hold the dental
dam in place and lick, lick, lick! Dental damns are so thin and sensual that she will feel plenty of sensation and the warmth of your
mouth.

If a dental dam in not available for you, you can use plastic wrap.
Yup. The same stuff you use in your kitchen to keep your food fresh.
Now you can use it while getting fresh with your lover! It's great
because you can use longer strips of it and not worry about it slipping away from your eager lips! Have your partner sit on the end of
it and unroll a large piece of it so that it's easy to hold the other end
in place. It's also see-through, which can help make your safer sex

---

HOMEWORK:

Be ready for hot sex.

- Shop for safer sex supplies like an optimist. Assume you are going to need lots of safer sex supplies! Stock up on essentials: condoms, lube, dental dams, and gloves.
- Put your hot sex supplies in the places you would like to have sex, like near your bed, in the bathroom, in your backpack, in your glove box, and in the kitchen drawer. This makes spontaneous sex more possible.
- Speak to your lover about safer sex long before you are ever naked. It is much easier to talk about safer sex with your clothes on.
- Get tested. Ask your lover to get tested. Take your best friend and get tested together. It is sometimes more comfortable getting tested if you have a friend there to hold your hand. Or if you prefer, there are clinics that will test you anonymously.
- If you stumble onto someone else's safer sex stash, don't make judgments on their behavior, laugh, or make fun of them. Instead applaud them for knowing how to care for themselves.

---

look more like oral sex should look like. Plus, plastic wrap now comes in all sorts of colors. I recommend using the nonmicrowavable plastic wrap, because if it's made to use in the microwave that means it is porous and not a suitable safer sex barrier.

When can a couple be certain about practicing unprotected sex?

Having unprotected sex can be an alluring thing. Direct skin-on-skin contact between you and your lover can wake up some of your deepest sexual instincts and enhance the feelings of intimacy. Regardless, unless you are trying to get pregnant, I do not recommend having unprotected sex. The smartest thing to do is care for yourself and your partner by having safer sex.

If you are insistent upon having unprotected sex, you and your lover should talk about the risks involved. Each of you should get thoroughly tested for STDs, and opposite sex couples need to consider pregnancy and birth control issues. Talk about what happens if one of you decides you want to go back to using latex barriers or if one of you decides no longer to be monogamous. If you are having unprotected sex with your partner and decide to have a sexual encounter outside of this relationship, be sure to practice safe sex in an effort to care for your primary partner.

Ask your doctor to test you for:

- Bacterial vaginosis (female, acquired through sex or unbalanced vaginal ecology)
- Chlamydia
- CMV
- Genital warts (HPV)
- Gonorrhea
- Hepatitis
- Herpes
- HIV

- Molluscum contagiosum
- Pelvic inflammatory disease (female, acquired through sex or unbalanced vaginal ecology)
- Syphilis
- Trichomoniasis

Perhaps these steps sound extreme, but it's so easy to pass simple bacteria infections. Humans have a history of making bad decisions and sometimes at the expense of someone they love. It is all too common for a partner of any gender to step outside of a bonded relationship and put their partner at risk.

Beyond that, in my lifetime I have seen HIV and AIDS take the lives of too many beautiful people. The more people practicing safer sex as a normal part of life, the fewer people to be infected and affected.

What Is Safer Sex?

Safer sex is simply sex with care. It means taking care of yourself and your lover(s). Having safer sex means reducing your risk of acquiring and/or spreading infections and diseases. Having safer sex also means protecting yourself or your partner from becoming pregnant. It's important to know this stuff because when you are feeling sexed up and acting on pure animal urges, it can be harder to practice safer sex than it sounds! It's good to read up and be prepared. That way when you are ready to get it on, you don't have to think much!

Having safer sex means using barriers (like condoms,

gloves, and dental dams) between you and your lover to avoid swapping fluids like vaginal fluids, semen, breast milk, and blood (including menstrual blood.) These barriers will protect your mouth, hands, vagina, penis, rectum, and sex toys from any sexually transmitted infections (STIs) or diseases (STDs). These STI/STDs can sound scary, but the truth is that people need sex. And you cannot know if a person has an STI/STD by looking at them. Lots of good, sweet, honest, decent people have contracted sexually transmitted infections and diseases. You need to be prepared. Learn to eroticize sexual barriers.

Some people fear that if a new lover discovers that they have a stash of sex supplies, it will reflect upon their character. Some people worry that it will make them look like a slut and others worry that their lover will assume they are a player. Wise up. A person who has safer sex supplies on hand is a responsible adult. They are ready to care for themselves and their lover and should be respected for it.

I have a nail-biting and cuticle-biting habit. Can I get sick or get an infection if I put my fingers inside my lover?

Yes. You are both at risk. Buy some smooth latex gloves. I recommend using them even if your hands are in good condition. Why not avoid introducing new bacteria into your lover's body from under your nails or possibly cutting delicate tissue with sharp fingernails? The better your gloves fit, the easier it will be for you to use your hands on your partner and the better they will feel. A well-fitting latex glove that is dripping with lube is a very sexy thing. And safe, too!

Why do some women get bladder infections after sex?

A woman's urethra opens up right near or actually inside a woman's vaginal opening. It is in fact nestled so close to the vaginal opening that bacteria from your vagina or partner can get pushed up into the opening of your urethra. For this reason I recommend going to pee immediately after sex (not just intercourse but any sex play that involves her vulva) to flush out your urethra.

13.

Her Orgasm: The Art & Science

When it comes to orgasmic response women report wild variations. One woman may find her orgasms to be elusive. Another woman may report having the subtlest tremors. And other women tell tales of muscle-pumping explosions. Speak to enough women and you will find every point in between. With female partners, each woman you encounter will be a new experience.

What exactly is a female orgasm?

An orgasm is a series of involuntary muscular contractions in the pelvis. The stronger your pelvis muscles are, the bigger your orgasm will be.

How do you know if you are having an orgasm?

Sometimes it can be hard for a woman to know. If you have never had one before or if your muscles are not too strong, it may be a subtle sensation. An orgasm can feel like a couple of quick twinges or a series of powerful muscular surges that reverberate through your pelvis and thighs. If you want to explore how to make your orgasms stronger, review the Chapter 6 instructions on how to strengthen your pelvis muscles.

Are there different types of female orgasms?

Although all orgasms are defined as a series of muscular contractions there are a number different ways you can set off these contractions. The most common way a female can reach orgasm is through stimulating her clit. Other women will be inspired to orgasm by having their g-spot stimulated. And still other women will have their orgasms sparked by consciously or unconsciously engaging and flexing their muscles. Any combination of these techniques may work as well. Some women find they need to tense up their muscles to orgasm, while other women need to be very relaxed. These various techniques for orgasming and the fact that much of the female sexual anatomy is internal and not visible can make it difficult for a woman to understand how and why she can or cannot orgasm. It can become more or less complex with age, because as a woman grows and changes in life she may find new responses and new ways to inspire orgasms.

Is it difficult or impossible for some women to have an orgasm?

It can be difficult to orgasm. Sure. It can involve using your fingers and/or sex toys to wake up nerve endings and expand neural pathways.

At the same time you'll need to work to engage your muscles, breathe, and become more conscious of your body. This not an instant process for many women; it requires lots of practice and patience. You may have numerous experiences where you feel very excited but cannot seem to tip yourself over the edge. Learning to orgasm can be totally frustrating, but don't give up!

Other women let insecurities or fears inhibit their ability to fully enjoy sex. For example, some women fear they will wet the bed during sex or they may become obsessed with some perceived imperfection on their body. They can become so sidetracked with theses thoughts that they cannot enjoy sex.

There are indeed women who cannot orgasm. Some instances where women may not be able to orgasm include instances where she has damaged her clit in an accident or some other pelvic trauma, she may have a disease that affects her nervous and/or muscular system, or she may be disabled in some other way.

In many cases a woman who has limited or no clitoral sensation can work to engage her pelvic muscles and learn to orgasm. Doing the pelvic muscle exercises outlined in Chapter 6 will only benefit any woman who seeks to strengthen her orgasm or orgasm for the first time. If your partner is disabled in any way, don't underestimate her sexuality. All a person really needs in order to be sexual is a nice juicy brain. The explorations a woman's mind can take her on are far more expansive than any series of muscular contractions!

How can I achieve an orgasm?

For most women the best way to explore orgasmic response is to do it alone. That way you can direct all of your focus on your body and orgasmic response without the distraction of having to interact with or please your partner. Try to set aside an hour or so just for you to explore your body and your orgasmic response. You may try these tips and orgasm on your first attempt or you may need to patiently explore your body for a month or two.

1) Spoil yourself. Buy some sexy accoutrements like lube, a quality deep-tissue vibrating massager, bubble bath, erotic books, videos, or anything else that piques your sexual interest.

2) Find a comfortable and quiet place. Set yourself up in a comfortable position. Most people like to be on their back, possibly with a pillow or two behind them and their legs spread comfortably. Other people like to lie on their belly. You might even like to play in the bathtub.

3) Put a little lube on your vulva. If you plan on using your fingers or toy internally be sure to put a little lube on your vaginal opening as well.

4) Let your mind wander to any thoughts that may turn you on. Remember that your imagination is yours to play with. Think about a past sexual experience or something you have never tried before. There are no forbidden sexual thoughts. If you would like some inspiration I recommend reading *My Secret Garden*, by Nancy Friday. This book is full of real women's sexual fantasies. It may help

you dream up new fantasies or help you recognize how normal and natural it is to have perverse sexual thoughts. You could also read other erotica books or watch adult movies for inspiration. If your thoughts wander away from what you are doing or your sex fantasy, just gently guide it back to your last racy thought. Staying focused is not always easy.

5) Let your hands linger over your pussy. Use a few fingers to tap on your clit. Let your fingers glide through your soft pussy lips. Dip your fingers inside your vagina if that feels good to you. Put a little pressure on your perineum, always returning to your clit to stroke, rub, or tap. By doing this you are waking up your nerves and bringing more blood circulation into your pussy.

6) As your fingers move over your pussy start to gently flex your pelvic muscles in a rhythmic fashion or rock your pelvis back and forth. Let your breath get deeper, taking in as much air as is comfortable for you. Your goal is to pull as much blood and oxygen into your pelvic muscles as you possibly can. Breathing through your sex play is very important. Breathing provides the oxygen you need to get the optimal use of your muscles.

7) Once you are feeling more sensation in your pelvis, use your fingers or your vibrating massager directly on or near your clit. Continue to flex your muscles and breathe. You

may have a few minutes of a plateau here or there. That's
normal. Do this as long as it feels good.

8) If this does not work the first few times, continue to
   explore and expand the kinds of play you engage in.
   Change positions. Try a new sex toy. Put a toy inside your
   pussy. Go back to using your fingers. Scoot your pussy
   under the bathtub faucet and let the water splash on your
   pussy. Use your showerhead. There is no right way or
   wrong way to touch yourself.

How can I guarantee an orgasm during sex?

You can't. It is the rare person who orgasms every single time they
have sex. That does not mean that sex does not feel good, it's just
that sometimes our bodies do not go there. The best thing you can
do is let your partner know. You could say something like, "Mmmm
. . . This feels good. . . . But I don't think I am going to orgasm
tonight." This way they are not running themselves ragged as they
try to get you somewhere you may not want to or can't go that night.
If your partner seems upset by this, pull them in close and let them
know you love their body and sharing yourself with them. And partners: please don't get upset or blame yourself if sometimes your
partner does not orgasm. It's normal.

How can you tell if a woman is faking an orgasm?

You can't always tell. Some women are very good at faking. If she is
faking it is usually because she is too insecure to share how she really
needs to be touched and does not want to hurt your feelings. Or

perhaps she does not know how to orgasm or has never orgasmed during partner play or penetration alone.

Rather than trying to catch her faking, you would be better off working to open up your lines of communication when it comes to sex. Start by speaking in positives around sex. Tell her if she does something that feels really good. Give her an honest compliment on her body or abilities. Talk about sex after a fun bout of sex play; talk about sex at times when neither one of you is naked. The more trust she has with you the easier it will be for her to tell you the truth about her body and her response.

Ask her to show you how she touches herself. Watch what she does and learn how to touch her! Give her a vibrator and encourage her to use it alone and during partner play. When having sex together, tune in to the subtle changes in her body as she experiences different levels of excitement. Listen to her breath. Watch her chest rise and fall. If she is breathing shallow, then ask her to breathe for you. (That's hot!) If you are inside her, see if you can feel her muscles work around your fingers or penis. If you can't, then ask her to flex them for you. Become engaged with her body and help her become engaged with it as well. Watch her hips rise or fall with various touches. Listen to the noises she makes. If she seems to "check out" during sex, see if you can catch a little eye contact with her so she knows you are present.

If she has been faking orgasms it may be difficult or impossible for her to tell you. But if she does, let her know she is safe with you and that you are sincerely ready to help her find her orgasms. It's a big step for a woman to fess up to faking and can lead the two of you on to very exciting and fun new places together.

FACT:

According to a study cited in Dr. Ruth's *Sex for Dummies,* lesbians have more orgasms than heterosexual women. They speculate this is because lesbians tend to arouse each other more slowly and communicate more during sex, telling each other more explicitly what is sexually pleasing.

How normal is it for a woman to need to be touched on her clit in order to orgasm?

It's totally normal. Studies show that less than 30 percent of women can orgasm from penetration alone. If you need to have clit stimulation to orgasm you are normal. Please don't hesitate to touch yourself during sex. It is so *sexy* when a woman touches herself! If you look at sexual imagery of women, like in movies or on television, women are always running their hands along their thighs or across their necks. It is sexy and sensual when a woman touches herself.

If your partner needs to touch herself in order to orgasm don't take it as an insult to your skills. This is just how her body is built, and she is normal. Instead encourage her to touch herself. Enjoy the show! Watch what she does and learn how to touch her. Give her a vibrator and encourage her to use it during sex. Watch how she uses it and learn how to touch her!

Get it? Ladies, it's up to you to be open to sharing how you get off; and, partners, it's up to you to learn how to touch her. It's that simple.

> **FACT:**
>
> According to Kinsey the average time it takes for a women to attain orgasm by way of masturbation is four minutes.

Is a clitoral orgasm really different from a vaginal orgasm?

Every orgasm, no matter how it is triggered, is a series of muscular contractions. How extreme the orgasm is depends upon how strong her muscles are. The clit is the easiest way, and for many women the only way, to trigger these orgasmic contractions. For some women, having her g-spot stimulated will inspire enough sensation and pressure to cause orgasmic muscular contractions. Other women will pump their muscles during solo or partner play, and that alone may pull enough blood and oxygen into her pelvis to cause orgasmic muscular contractions. Or she may use any combination of these techniques to stir up an orgasm.

Depending upon how she triggers her orgasm, these contractions may feel different. Most often I hear clitoral-triggered orgasms feel higher pitched. The contractions tend to be short bursts. While orgasms driven by pumping her muscles will feel more deep and drawn out. Of course every woman is unique. How orgasms feel for each woman is relevant to her body alone.

True Tales of Female Orgasms:

"I enjoy my orgasms more when my partner helps me (through penetration with either his hands or penis) but I find it takes me longer to climax when he is around than when I do it alone. Alone it can take me under five minutes, if even that, depending on my mood, and with him it can go on for up to thirty minutes and sometimes I just give up."

"I've never been able to have an orgasm during sex with a man, with just penetration. I like the feeling of penetration most times and I really wish I could cum at the same time, but I haven't been able to so far without the help of a vibrator."

"I've had some mega-intense orgasms through masturbation, but they are always really short and intense, and very utilitarian. With my partner, who I've been with for three years, they are just an entirely different thing, in the 'oh my god, toe curling, I think I am going to end up with a charlie horse' type way where they last for much longer, and I can feel them much more in the entirety of my body. It's really amazing."

"So far, I have only been able to have clitoral orgasms. Using my hand or my lover's tongue. I guess humping something also works. When I discovered the Hitachi Magic Wand, my world was changed and I was finally able to have multiple orgasms. The most I had in a row (yes, I counted because it

was such a surreal experience for me!) was forty-four. I find
that after ten orgasms it can get really 'spiritual' for lack of a
better word. I've tried to have an orgasm with my g-spot. So
far I haven't been successful but I'll keep trying!"

"I'm a clit girl all the way. Penetration feels really, really good
and so can g-spotting, but I don't orgasm without clit stimulation. Although there have been a few times that I've come
damn close just from someone skillfully sucking my nipples.
All this talk is making me randy."

"There's definitely nothing like good oral sex. It's just a heavenly feeling when done well. I think what makes an orgasm
feel more intense for me usually has psychological roots. If
I'm with a partner and they're talking dirty and being rough
in the ways that I like, that usually means I get really hot, thus
intense orgasm. On my own, I feel like my more intense
orgasms happen when I'm fantasizing about a new lover or
potential lover, replaying hot moments we've shared, etc."

"With masturbation there's no thought at all—I orgasm very
quickly. With my guy I have to work hard to keep my mind
turned off from wandering to thoughts about laundry, what I
forgot to do today, or how I feel fat and keep my mind on the sexy
things going on. But it's much better when sparks finally fly."

"I'm definitely a clit girl. Stimulation by hand is great (index
and middle finger of the right hand, to be specific.) Certain

toys are good. Most vibes are too intense for me but there are a few that are 'throbby' instead of 'buzzy' and they definitely get the job done. And a well-trained lover's tongue is probably my favorite tool of all."

" When I masturbate, my orgasms tend to be quick and very intense. Just your basic 'get off and get on with your day' sort of thing. But my partner-play orgasms are much longer lasting and more interesting. I am particularly fond of being orally stimulated almost to orgasm and then penetrated forcefully and vigorously. That usually results in a toe-curling, eyes-rolled-back-in-the-head, bed-shaking, screaming orgasm that lasts for several minutes. **"**

"I give myself very good, quick orgasms when I need to, but my boyfriend has given me a new perspective. I never really had orgasms very well with anyone before him. He takes his time, has the most amazing tongue. And while I haven't come strictly from penetration, he gives me a combo of clitoral stimulation and dirty talking, and I explode into a divine feeling that lasts for almost ten-fifteen minutes afterward. It's not like when I am alone, though. With him it seems like I really have to set my mind to it and force myself to relax and let go and let the sex conquer all."

"When I masturbate, my best orgasms are sparked by a combination of clitoral play and internal massage lightly over the g-spot. What I love is using my detachable showerhead to provide constant stimulation of my clitoris while I use my middle finger and index finger of my right hand to massage around and on both sides of my g-spot. I have a short vagina so the g-spot is not very far in. While with a male partner, I prefer some type of pressure on my clitoris or I rarely reach an orgasm. Since manual stimulation usually takes a long time for me to reach an orgasm (at least twenty minutes), I prefer to hump something, be it the corner of a chair, or a pillow with my hand between it and me."

"When I was younger, it was solely external clitoral. As I became more comfortable with my sexuality and increased exploration and self-awareness, I began experiencing internal g-spot orgasms. Now I love the fact I can experience various combinations. I used to prefer being on top of my partner just for the clitoral stimulation, but now it's more for the internal."

"I didn't buy a toy until I was in my early thirties, after a friend's recommendation. After my first week of playing with it, I finally confronted her—shook her by the shoulders, and said '*Why* didn't you convince me to buy a vibrator long before now!' "

"My masturbation orgasms are typically quick and intense, but not 'deep.' I usually enjoy partner play more, because of the element of anticipation and surprise—seeming not to have control."

What is the best way to stimulate the g-spot?

The g-spot is on the navel side of her vaginal wall and about one and a half to two inches inside her vagina. The best way to stimulate it is with fingers. Due to the positioning of the g-spot in her body it can be nearly impossible for a woman to stimulate her own g-spot with her fingers. So, partners, it's up to you! Once you have warmed her up a bit (think oral sex, sex toys . . .), insert one or two fingers up to about the second knuckle. Instead of doing an in-and-out motion, what you need to do is a massage—pushing or rubbing on her g-spot area or doing a "come here" sort of motion with your fingers. Sometimes it helps to use your other hand to put pressure on her clit or even to push down on her pubic bone from the outside of her body while your other hand is working her from the inside.

14.

His Orgasm:
The Art & Science

M en are much deeper and far more sexually beautiful than the world gives them credit for. Sure, the bulk of their sexual anatomy is easy to see and touch, but their brain, nerves, and blood vessels are complex and unique to each individual. Frequently women will ask me for a simple "tip that is sure to blow his mind!" and guys will ask for fresh, new ideas for how to touch themselves and bring on bigger or different kinds of orgasms. Once again I say, orgasm is art. If you have male partners, each man you encounter will be a new experience.

What techniques do you recommend to stimulate a man to orgasm?

Most guys want specific kind or kinds of rhythmic sensations to bring them to orgasm. The sensation that will bring your guy to orgasm will be unique to him. The very best way to learn how to bring him to orgasm is to watch him give himself an orgasm. This can be a tough thing to ask a guy to do if you are shy or if he is self-conscious, but it can be very exciting for both of you! If you are shy it may be easier for you to sit behind him while he masturbates for you. This way the both of you can watch the action without the pressure of having to look each other in the eye. (Unless that turns you on!) I also like doing this from behind him because you get to see how he touches himself from his perspective. Watch where he places his hand, how his speed or pressure may change. Watch what he does and steal his moves!

There are lots of other little things you can do like stroking or licking his balls, cupping his balls, massaging his perineum, or flicking your tongue around and under the head of his penis. Experiment. If you are trying something new ask him, "Does this feel good? Harder? Faster? Softer?" If you are in the middle of sex play try to ask yes-or-no questions so that he can communicate with you without having to go into deep explanations. Watch his hips, his breath, and listen for little noises. All of these things will clue you in to how he is responding to your touch.

What is the best way to handle a guy who is having a difficult time getting it up?

With kindness and the understanding that not being able to get an erection is a normal obstacle that many men face at some point in their lives. Most often it means he may have something he needs to address in his life—physical or emotional. Think of it as a call to consciousness. His body is asking the two of you to slow down and look at the bigger picture.

A rather large percentage of men who have trouble getting or maintaining an erection suffer from diseases like diabetes, kidney disease, back problems, alcoholism, or clogged arteries. However, not being able to keep an erection isn't necessarily an indicator he is experiencing one of these ailments. Bu if his erection trouble appear to be chronic, you could make an appointment with your doctor and run a few tests for any of the diseases I have mentioned. (Check out Chapter 12 for information on how to find a sex-positive doctor.)

Other leading causes include anxiety, stress, and depression. If he is able to get an erection in his sleep, then his trouble is very likely caused by something that is pressing him emotionally. It never hurts to sit down and make an action list of the things that may by stressing you out and one thing you can do under each item to help reduce that stress. Solo and couples counseling may also be a great way to assess and resolve emotional issues.

While you are working to improve his life conditions, try to concentrate on sex play that is not orgasm focused. Give each other massages, take baths together, have movie dates, enjoy sex play in any way your bodies may take you. Just because you do not orgasm does not mean the touch and interactions do not feel good. With a little attention and patience most people find their erections again.

What can you do to keep a guy's erection while using a condom?

You may want to experiment with different kinds of condoms. The condom you are using may be too tight or too big. Plus now there are oodles of great condoms on the market. Condoms with more room at the tip so he can get more blood circulation in that area, condoms with textures on the inside and some condoms that feel so thin that guys report the need to continually check to see if it is still on. Most pharmacies are not going to have the best collection of condoms. Check out the Resources section at the back of this book for a list of quality retailers.

Before you put the condom on him put a drop or two of lube inside the condom. This will create a feeling of wetness to go with the warmth of your body.

Sometimes we make the problem only worse when we apologize for needing to use condoms or start to demonize them. Although it's not always easy try to eroticize condoms. Start by putting a positive spin on condoms. For example, the next time you want to have sex, hand him a condom and ask him, "Do you wanna get some?" Essentially you are using the condom to flirt! Anytime you speak of condoms try to do it in a happy, light way. Ultimately you want him to start to associate condoms with fun.

True Tales of Male Orgasms:

"The best orgasms I've ever had have all been from blowjobs. As much as I enjoy intercourse, it's far too easy to climax quickly, and that puts a damper on how much I (and she) enjoy the experience. The best way to get me off? Start with a hand job/blowjob, switch to intercourse, and finish off with more oral sex. This generally leaves me so worked up that I can't stop shaking for ten minutes afterward. Orgasms from masturbation are far more direct and far less enjoyable. I know exactly what I like and so it's very easy to come, but there's nothing too special or unique about doing it. Right now I'm going through a hand-job phase, where I really love to have my cock handled and pulled on and tugged on, but before that I was going through an oral phase where that was really what I was wanting. It's normal for me to go through phases like that."

"I get to the point of orgasm much quicker during intercourse, but if my girlfriend is giving me head, when I finally do come it feels much, *much* better. Like lose-all-control-and-have-violent-muscle-spasms better. She definitely knows how to get me worked up nice and slowly."

"My most satisfying solo orgasms are nothing compared to the first time my girlfriend gave me the first of many hand jobs. I was lying on my back and was rather nervous (which may have helped me not ejaculate prematurely), but forty-odd minutes later I came so ferociously it startled her and she bent my penis backwards. I wound up shooting my wad over my own head (it landed on a bookshelf a foot or so away), and I spent several minutes afterward uncontrollably quivering and giggling while trying to apologize for getting goo on her possessions."

"My orgasms happen the quickest from masturbation, and can be quite intense but not as wracking as the lengthy buildup I experience when orgasming during sex with my partner. My most powerful orgasms come from vaginal intercourse during, or just after, fetish or BDSM play. Orgasms from vaginal intercourse take a long time to happen for me, as if they have to be dragged from my brain, but when they do happen they are senses-shattering. The more intense and kinky the scene before intercourse, the faster I orgasm. Anal stimulation from toys or fingers also speeds up and intensifies orgasms from either masturbation or vaginal sex. I usually don't come at all from anal or oral, despite my frequent enjoyment of both. I don't really know why."

"I can generally only achieve orgasm by my own hand. Sometimes receiving oral can get me over the top, but it takes a long time. I've learned over the years to deemphasize my own orgasm and just enjoy whatever act I'm engaged in on its own level. Then at the end of play, I enjoy having my lover embrace me while I bring myself to orgasm."

"I like to have my cock head concentrated on but I also enjoy the shaft stimulation. Lube is always good, but not too much, because then you lose the friction. I am not at all wild about having my balls played with. For me it just doesn't feel good. It makes me feel endangered, for some reason. And for some reason anal stimulation makes me lose my erection. I don't know whether that's psychological or what. There is a difference between masturbation orgasms and partner play orgasms for me. Masturbation orgasms can be extremely intense, but they can also be a bit, I guess, lonely, for lack of a better word. Partner orgasms feel different for me. There's more of an energy exchange going on, a wavelike exchange of energy (as corny as that may sound) that makes the orgasm feel bigger and more satiating."

"I'm all for technology in bed. A vibrator used on me can be fun, or it can just be annoying. I like some overall pressure as well as vibration. I've used a variety of cock rings. Any kind of constriction at the base is a recipe for more pressure, bigger, harder. It's also likely to maintain the erection for a bit after orgasm, but the sensation is so much more intense that I'm ready to stop right there. The remaining erection is pretty much just for show."

"I find the orgasms from vaginal intercourse to be the least exciting. They're good; I mean any orgasm is good. But probably the most intense ones are from a really good hand job. I suspect it's because the woman giving me one has much better control of her hands and their manipulation of me than if she were using another part of her body. A really, really good blowjob comes in close second. Ones from anal sex (giving or receiving) are pretty good, too, but I suspect that's mostly the psychological naughty factor. But my best orgasms are from an eager-to-please woman with a handful of lube and a gleam in her eye."

❝ Never underestimate the power of your tongue. Of course I'm talking about talking dirty during sex. It can totally push me over the edge if a girl starts talking really dirty while we're fucking. ❞

"Since my accident when I was paralyzed I never have been able to trigger an orgasm by any sexual encounter (penetration, hand, blowjob) that would physically be counted as such. I sort of achieve a 'mental orgasm'; for example, when my last girlfriend came by cunnilingus I somehow shared with her the feeling—afterward being relaxed and exhausted. Then I discovered that I could trigger a full physical orgasm with the massage shower in my last apartment. That was incredible—my first orgasm after five years was like the first one in life! It takes quite a bit of stimulus to trigger. It continued to be especially difficult to bring myself there until I bought a Hitachi Magic Wand two years ago. Works like a charm. But the interesting part is: with this I can trigger a full-blown physical orgasm (indeed several in a row; tried it up to 7 in 30 minutes), but I have to concentrate. Indeed I can have an orgasm without nearly any 'emotional response' at all."

"I've had mind-blowing, near-psychedelic orgasms both with my girlfriend and alone, and in several different ways. The thing I find most interesting about the different ways of reaching orgasm is how different they are. Not necessarily better or less good, but each most certainly has its own character. The one thing that the best ones have in common is a long, long buildup. Whether it means toying with myself while watching porn, or a long slow grind of intercourse, it's all about teasing and stopping, taking it to the brink and then falling back. Where the experience changes most is at the actual moment of orgasm. Masturbation is a pure sensual release, at its best a sort of meditation where, like in the psychedelic experience, momentary ego death is achieved and I feel at one with the universe upon climax. I know, it sounds crazy if you talk about it in the harsh light of day, but I have felt it many times. Orgasm through vaginal intercourse is the most bonding and spiritually loving sensation. When I come that way with my girlfriend, I feel closer to her than I have ever felt to anyone. The pleasure is intense, and the body is exhausted, but there is a feeling that I believe must be the diametric opposite of loneliness."

"My best orgasms tend to come after a long buildup, no matter how they're achieved. Each one is a little different for me, though. Receiving anal with penile stimulation gives me an all-over body release. I feel like I've had a good massage after those. The bigger the object (fists, butt plugs, etc.), the bigger the release. I also tend to be done after those orgasms. Vaginal and giving anal tend to be about the same. Great release, but I can also recover from them to have another orgasm. Masturbation tends to be a quick release. Sweet candy. It helps in the moment, but missing the extra component of a partner it tends to be less satisfying in the long run. Having someone share your arousal is a huge element of the turn-on for me."

How can I get him hard more than once in a night?

You may not be able to get him hard more than once in an evening. Young men can experience multiple erections with a certain amount of ease, but as men start climbing up into their thirties they tend to cool out a bit. Be careful not to compare your body or your lover's body to that of an eighteen-year-old. It can be hard on a guy's ego.

There is, however, one advantage some older men have (or can have) over younger men and that is better familiarity with their bodies. With a little work and discipline many men can become more conscious in their bodies and learn to open up their nerve connections with their pelvic muscles and orgasmic response.

There are a number of exercises he can do, including breathing, muscle flexing, and paying close attention to his orgasmic response so he can learn to separate the feelings of ejaculation from the feelings of orgasmic contractions. With practice he may be able to inspire multiple muscular orgasms (sometimes called dry orgasms) and delay his ejaculation. Some men can have sex for hours, letting their erection rise and subside throughout the night by using this method.

I recommend reading *The Multi-Orgasmic Man,* by Mantak Chia and Douglas Abrams, for in-depth instructions on expanding male orgasmic response.

FACT:

When a man is orgasming his breath can increase up to forty breaths per minute. The muscles at the base of his penis contract at 0.8-second intervals with intensity capable of squirting ejaculate up to two feet in distance.

What does it mean if your male partner takes forever to orgasm?

It is normal for many guys to take a "long time" to orgasm. Remember, what's a long time to one person may not be so long to another. Many men report the longer it takes, the more intense the orgasm is. I suggest you talk to him about why it takes him so long. Some guys have a great deal of control over how quickly they orgasm. If you let him know that you are tired, he may be able to orgasm at will and make the experience easier for you. You can also find ways to build your stamina. Using lubricant can cut down on friction and make longer bouts of intercourse a lot more pleasurable. Finding sexual positions that support your body will also help you feel better during sex. Use pillows to prop up your head, neck, tummy, butt, or back during sex play.

FACT:

According to *Playboy* magazine, with consistent rhythm, it takes 7.3 minutes for the average man to ejaculate. That number drops down to 1.8 minutes for men who struggle with early ejaculation.

How much fluid is to be expected from ejaculation exactly?

The average guy will ejaculate approximately a few teaspoons' worth of fluid. The quantity and texture can vary if he has had more than one orgasm that day. He may ejaculate more fluid if he drinks plenty of water and is well hydrated. If he has a healthy diet he will probably have increased production in seminal fluids as well. That old saying is true—you are what you eat!

15

Foreplay:
A New Definition

When I first started teaching sex to women in a workshop format I was surprised to hear them consistently plead for more talk about foreplay. Flirting. Kissing. Massage. Fingers. Mouths. Dirty talk. Toys. Women everywhere were asking why they don't receive more foreplay and how to inspire their lovers to give more foreplay?

The topic of foreplay was a little baffling to me at the time. It had not occurred to me that women were not receiving foreplay. It wasn't clear what exactly they were craving. Luckily I was still working at a women-owned sex toy shop called Babeland. One day I took a poll of my coworkers. I asked each woman, "What is foreplay? How would you define it?"

Interestingly, none of us could come up with a satisfying answer. Like me, my coworkers weren't as concerned with foreplay as were my workshop participants. Why weren't we talking about or asking for more foreplay? And why was the word foreplay barely even a part of our vocabulary?

After reconsidering my test group of coworkers, the answer became obvious: most of us were lesbians or had substantial relationships with women. Women who have sex with other women have a different definition of what sex is. Sex for us does not start or end with intercourse. Sex starts with all the little interactions like kisses, flirting, and conversations. Sex can be an orgasm that happens when your lover knows how to rub you the right way, even with your clothes on. Sex can happen with a sex toy, or a hand job, or a gifted mouth. Sex can be the look in your lover's eyes when she sucks the whipped cream off your fingers. Unlike so many straight couples and even gay men, sex is never just penetration.

President Bill Clinton showed a lack of sexual sophistication when he told the world that having oral sex with Monica Lewinsky was not by definition having "sexual relations" with her, just as many young people today and throughout history have thought that by having oral sex or anal sex rather than vaginal sex they could still be classified as virgins.

This lack of information actually has dangerous consequences because the number one way we are spreading STDs today is through oral sex. We do ourselves a disservice when we think about sex as just intercourse or behave as if sex starts and stops with intercourse.

At the same time that I was exploring the idea of foreplay I continued teaching and learning with men and women. These explicit conversations I have had with them have proven to me that the best lovers are men and women who are generous in bed. Their heads are not in their pants or panties. They're seeing a bigger picture. Those are the people who find pleasure in seeing their partner excited and orgasming. They ask questions and use everything available to them to help make sex hotter.

Why don't the men I have encountered understand that foreplay is a very important part of a sexual encounter?

It is a combination of factors that lead people (men and women) to believe that sex is all about intercourse. For example, religious groups have long taught that sex is for procreation and any pleasure found outside of this act is sinful. It is also the misguided teachings of leading medical professionals like Sigmund Freud, who contended that the clitoral orgasm was adolescent, and that upon puberty, when women begin having intercourse with men, she should transfer the center of orgasm to the vagina.

Our cultural leaders continue to perpetuate these ideas because our society is full of myths about sex, preferring instead to keep all of us in the dark. It is up to you to teach your lovers how to touch you. Inspire them to read books and learn with you. It is up to you to provide quality sex education to your children as well. Find age-appropriate books to share with them as they mature. You can find a few of the books I recommend in the Resources section at the back of this book.

— : — : —

True Tales of Foreplay:

"I love foreplay. It's my favorite part of sex. The kissing, the touching, the searching. And giggling. Good foreplay has lots of giggling!"

"Foreplay is kissing kissing kissing kissing, biting, scratching, spanking, staring into each other's eyes with wicked grins and wrestling to see who gets to be the dominant one and who gets to be the submissive! Sometimes foreplay (if lucky) is also writing each other deliciously deviant letters or E-mails or talking on the phone. Do I wish for more foreplay? Heck ya. For *me*, foreplay is the best part."

"For me, foreplay includes all the touching, rubbing, binding, masturbating, oral play, anal (digital) play, snuggling, nibbling, whispering that can go on! If you can add an 'ing' on to it, it could be some type of foreplay."

"I like biting/sucking/kissing on my neck, ass smacks/ squeezes, and scratches. Sex is defined for me as intercourse and oral, and starts when either happens."

"There are as many definitions of foreplay as there are people who enjoy it. It's something as simple as catching each other's eyes, or as complicated as intricate rope bondage. It is the fine art of titillation."

❝ The 'when does foreplay end and sex start' question is a lot like the 'chicken and egg' question. You can argue it a multitude of ways and make it sound good. Sex starts when you feel like it starts. And for me, that's different from time to time. There's an implication that sex starts when you cross some 'invisible line.' Where I draw that line differs from day to day. **❞**

"My favorite thing to do during foreplay is to have my inner elbow licked, sucked. and nibbled on. . . . And almost better than oral sex is licking, sucking, and nibbling on my hips. . . . Total yum!"

"My favorite foreplay is rough, like horseplay. Hair tugging, skin biting. The sweet taste of fresh sweat. The game is exploration and a struggle. Sex begins as a transgression and ends as a union. I love looking around the room, once my attention again can look beyond the world of my lover, and surveying the destruction. Mattress overturned and on the floor. The lingering question—'Where are my pants?' "

"I took a class on human sexuality. We had gone through the textbook 'classical' stage of intercourse. The question was asked, 'When does foreplay start?' The professor didn't blink an eye. 'Foreplay starts when you say, "So how was your day?"' Her point was that foreplay is more of a psychological mindset than any specific actions. I have always remembered that. Sometimes someone will innocently ask me about my day and I will start giggling!"

"Sam Kinison, the comedian, used to say, 'Make her cum twice before she even sees your dick.' It's been my experience that, indeed, lots of foreplay and giving her an orgasm or two before I even get my belt undone makes quite the impression."

How do you get someone to kiss you without slobbering all over you? How do you get them to kiss more gently?

You need to guide them gently and lead by example. The next time your partner leans in to slobber on you, stop them just before they meet your lips and say, "I want to show you the kind of kiss I have been dreaming of." And then lay it on them. Ask them to do it back to you. Make it fun.

It is so easy to tell a person what *not* to do. If they kiss you in a sloppy way or touch you in a way that hurts, you might say, "Ouch!" or "Please don't do that." This is appropriate in some situations, but not a productive way to get what your really want. If you only tell them what you don't want, they only know what not to do. No matter what kind of sex play you are having, try to speak to them in positives.

If they respond to your kissing demonstration by kissing back gently, tell them. "I like that, your lips are soft. But now again but not so wet." This advice applies to acts beyond kissing. If they use their fingers on your shaft in a way you like, tell them. If they held your leg in just the right position during intercourse, tell them! This is a great way to get what you want and have your lover feel like they are pleasing you.

Where do you start with foreplay?

You probably already know where to start. If you can, think back to the kind of sexual fun you may have been having before you were having penetrative play. (By penetrative play I mean oral sex, vaginal sex, or anal sex.) Think back to your first boyfriend or girlfriend. Remember what it was like to have long make-out session, complete with hot and heavy petting? Flirting, kissing, groping, knee humping, fingers, heart racing, sex through your clothes. For many guys, the kind of sex play that would stir up your sexual anticipation until you felt like you were going to explode. That could be fun or it could leave you in a frenzy of wanting. For a lot of women heavy petting alone can be very hot sex. But as we mature sexually we learn that this slow buildup can deliver explosive orgasms for everyone involved.

The next time you have sex with your partner, try to slow down. Leave your clothes on for an extra ten minutes and see how excited you can get each other through your clothing. When you do undress, set another allotment of time where the two of you will play without penetration of any kind. Let your fingers do the walking. Kiss. Laugh. Slow down and see where it takes you.

HOMEWORK:

Sloppy, sticky food foreplay is fun! Slathering yourself and your lover in cake, honey, whipped cream, cookie dough, chocolate syrup, or ice cream can be a blast! But if you are a woman, or having sex with a woman, it's important to remember that sugar should not go inside her vagina. For some women sugar can throw off her natural Ph balance and lead to infection. And everyone knows a vaginal infection will ruin all your fun.

Also, remember that any foods that have oils in them should not come in contact with your latex safer sex materials. Oils break down latex, making your condom less effective. (Read labels. For example, whipped cream has oil in it.)

Now that you know what not to do, here's what to do. Get inspired. Go to the grocery store and shop with your lover. Rent the classic food sex film *9 1/2 Weeks* and watch it together. Slather that sweet sticky stuff everywhere! (Avoiding her vagina. You can still add drops to her clit and lick them off before they drip down.) Eat your desert off your lover's inner thighs, chest, or neck. Have your food play in the shower so you can wash off with soap before you use latex. Get messy! Have fun! It's good for you.

16.

Fingers, Hands, & Hand Jobs: Melts in Your Hands

L et me be the first to remind you how sexy your hands can be. It's true.

I remember the days when I worked a service industry job. I stood on one side of the counter while the customer stood on the other. Frequently the customer would have a sheet of paper in their hands which I would have to examine, allowing me to see their hands up close.

Once while standing at that counter, waiting for the next bombardment of customers, I confessed to a female coworker that I frequently entertained myself by checking out people's hands. She admitted that hands were a turn-on to her, too! Since then I have spoken with hundreds of women and men who agree.

You can tell a lot about a person by looking at their hands. My favorites are clean, strong hands. I like hands that are big enough to envelop my hand, can hold on tight, deliver a good smack, with smooth nails that can move through my most sensitive parts without scratching me, and most of all, frequently washed hands. (I'm into hygiene, what can I say?) Never underestimate the power of a manicure.

Hands are your most versatile sex tools. They are your "Plan B" when your partner is still going but your tired mouth or pussy needs a break. They can create excellent rhythm in their strokes. Tickling, rubbing, slapping, massaging, pinching, pulling, holding, stroking, grabbing, groping. . . . You name it, your hand can do it!

How to Give Her a Great Hand Job

- Look at your hands. Are they clean? Are they soft? Are they free of any scrapes or cuts? Are your nails smooth and short? Wash them if possible.
- Take off any bulky or sharp rings.
- Consider wearing latex gloves. It may not sound sexy, but a well-fitting, lubed-up latex glove is one of the softest and most sensual sensations ever!
- Use lube on your fingers. It feels good and helps protect her body from getting friction burns or microscopic tears that can leave her more vulnerable to bacterial infections or sexually transmitted diseases.
- She is the person who is the most familiar with her body and how she likes to be touched. During your hand play ask her yes-or-no questions to find out if what you are doing feels good, if she would like it faster, slower, harder, deeper, etc.

- The outside of her body is also very sensitive. Touching her vulva and clit will do amazing things for her.
- Go slow. Start by gently cupping your hand over her whole vulva. Use all four fingers to gently make circles around her clit. Slow moves will build her anticipation and give you plenty of opportunity to watch her response to the sensation so you can assess if you are going in the right direction.
- Tap on her pubic mound and clit. This will cause vibrations that may warm her up.
- Ask her to show you how she likes to be touched. Watch what she does and learn from her. If she is too shy, put your hand on her vulva and put her hand over your hand while you ask her to guide your touch.
- Try putting a finger inside her. And move it gently in and out. Ask her if she would like it faster or slower.
- Try using both hands, one rubbing her clit and the other fingering her vagina. You can also move your finger around while inside her in a gentle "come here" kind of movement, with your fingers pointed toward her navel.
- During any kind of sex play you can use your hands to explore her response. Run them over her chest, belly, inner thighs, through her hair or any spot that presents itself. Who knows what kind of erogenous zones you may discover?

I feel like I have become so used to orgasming with my boyfriend's fingers on my clit that I don't think I can come any other way. Any suggestions?

You are in a rut. This can happen to any of us. Humans, by nature, are lazy creatures, so when we find something that works we tend to rely on that one thing. As soon as you recognize that you are feeling too dependent on any one technique you should change it up. It may be a little frustrating the first few times, but you can reintroduce other techniques into your play. For example, try using your own fingers, penetrative play, or a sex toy, all while flexing your pelvic muscles and breathing.

True Tales of Hand Sex:

"Nothing. Beats. A hand job. In my book, anyway. I do believe it is my favorite act to give and receive, because it's so easy to give and receive at the same time!"

❝ I use my hands as much as possible. Since I am disabled and can control only about half my arm muscles and none of my fingers I do this very carefully. I keep my fingernails cut short, because otherwise a person can easily hurt the tender inner parts, especially me since I move the hand as a whole and not the fingers. As always imagination is helpful, since I have feeling in only parts of my hands and fingers (luckily I got enough imagination). **❞**

"Fingers, hands, and toes, when used correctly, can get me off—no penetration required."

"I don't like guys using their hands on my girly parts. Too much negative association. . . . Plus, they never do it right. Handling my breasts is rather nice and fun, though."

"In my twenties my big thing was body massage. I'd start at the little toes and do every single muscle up to the top of the head and back down again. Not unusual to take a couple of hours and a few times quite a bit longer. My dates got very relaxed—I think a couple orgasmed in their sleep. For me it was entirely the joy of taking the time to make a friend feel really nice. I like the feel of warm flesh under my hands and how it responds to pressure and friction."

"I *love* the 'come hither' motion. Palms facing the ceiling, two fingers inserted into the vagina and a smoothly executed 'come hither' motion finds my g-spot so fast."

When you are giving a hand job, why does the guy get so sensitive after they orgasm?

He gets erect when the muscles at the base of his penis relax and allow blood to flow into the chambers in his penis. As soon as he orgasms the blood very quickly retreats from those chambers. For guys this can feel like the pins-and-needles feeling many of us experience after our foot falls asleep. If your guy experiences this sensation he's OK. Just let him be for a few minutes until the blood flow balances out in his penis.

What is the best technique for a hand job?

The easiest technique is almost always going to be the technique your guy has been using all his life. The best way to figure out what that technique is, is to inspire him to show you. The next time you want to give him a hand job, ask him to show you how he likes it. If he's not too shy, he will.

If you are a couple who enjoys showing off and watching, this will be easy and fun. If not, it might be easier to do this if you sit behind him, let him lean back against you while he does his thing. In this position you will get to see how he touches himself from his perspective, and he gets to masturbate for you without the pressure of seeing you watch him.

If he is so shy that touching himself in front of you is not possible, put your hand on his shaft, take one of his hands and put it over your hand. Then ask him to guide your hand. The goal is to get him to tell you or show you exactly how he likes it. He is the only person who knows the best technique for his body.

This is a little hand-job technique that gets past women. Usually when we see the first sign of ejaculation we stop pumping. One thing guys frequently tell me is that when they give themselves hand jobs and they are about to orgasm, they will make sure to keep their hand on their shaft and moving until the orgasm is complete. These last three or four strokes can be some of the most satisfying stokes, but women tend to drop his cock like he's spurting hot lava or something! Keep your hand on his cock and give him the grand finale if that is something he enjoys.

I have heard that twisting your hand during a hand job is a good technique. What do you think?

Sure. For some guys. It may turn him on and get him harder. Other guys might find a twisting sensation to be irritating or an obstacle to getting the kind of rhythm they require to orgasm. It's all about his body. Any hand-job techniques I describe or that you see or hear about from other sources should be seen as inspiration. It is possible that your lover may respond to these touches, or he may have touches that are all his own.

Try adding a twist to your technique. You could also try:

- Praying Hands. Put your hands on either side of his shaft as if you have them folded in prayer. Simply press them together a little and rub up and down.
- OK Rings. With both hands press your index finger to your thumb to create the international OK sign. Wrap the rings you have created with your fingers and thumbs around his shaft and move them up and down to create a milking stroke.
- Sensation Play. Many guys have told me they enjoy feeling different soft textures on their cock. Guys have reported using things like pasta, cotton balls, silk panties, feather dusters, and saran wrap in conjunction with their hand job just to experience a different kind of sensation. It may sound funny but, if he's into it, it's really just harmless fun. Learn to play with him!

Generally speaking, the more exotic hand-job techniques will probably get him excited and pull more pressure into his penis, while the straightforward, long, rhythmic strokes will probably bring him to orgasm.

Can you explain how I can use my hands on his balls?

Try cupping his balls in your hand and gently pushing them up against his body. Massage them by rolling them around in your hand. Some guys may want a stronger touch, like pulling or twisting. But always progress slowly with any touches so you can watch his response and check in with him.

How to Give Him a Great Hand Job

- Use lube on your hands. Guys frequently use lube when they give themselves hand jobs because it creates the kind of friction that may feel good to them. Experiment with different kinds of lube and different amounts and explore which ones feel best for him. Try a thicker lube like Slippery Stuff, a thinner lube like Astroglide, and maybe a silicone lube like Eros.

- He is the person who is the most familiar with his body and how he likes to be touched. During your hand job ask him yes-or-no questions to find out if what you are doing feels good, if he would like it faster, slower, more pressure, less pressure, etc.

- Ask him to show you how he likes to be touched. Watch what he does and learn from him. If he is too shy, put your hand on his penis and put his hand over your hand while you ask him to guide your touch.

- During any kind of sex play you can use your hands to explore his response. Run them over his chest, belly, inner thighs, through his hair or any spot that presents itself. Who knows what kind of erogenous zones you may discover?

I have always avoided giving hand jobs on the theory that guys can do it to themselves better. Is that true?

Your hand job will never compare to the kind of hand job he can give himself. After all he has probably been giving himself hand jobs for years. Plus we are talking about a part of *his* body; he has a direct connection to his own nerves and muscles.

But there is no way he can create the kind of spontaneity that comes with a lover's touch. There is excitement just in the idea that he does not know what is going to happen next. Never underestimate the power of your touch. Put your hands on him, tune in to his response, ask him questions, and see where it takes you.

17

Oral Sex:
Melts in Your Mouth

Oral sex means using your mouth to stimulate your lover's body. More specifically it means using your mouth on their vulva or penis.

Oral sex is one of the sex acts that America's antiquated laws restrict. For some reason the religious types who ran early America thought that any sexual interaction that could not possibly produce a child was a crime. Oral sex (heterosexual or homosexual) is still against the law in Alabama, Arizona, Florida, Idaho, Kansas, Louisiana, Massachusetts, Minnesota, Mississippi, Georgia, North and South Carolina, Oklahoma, Oregon, Rhode Island, Utah, Virginia, and Washington, D.C. The real crime is when people try to police what consenting adults enjoy doing in the privacy of their own homes. These archaic laws make me want to pucker up and go on a cross-country crime spree!

What tips can I give my lover in order to get good oral sex?

Tell them the truth. Be as explicit as you can. Studies show the more explicit you can be in describing what you enjoy, the more orgasms you will have. Speak in positives. If they do something right, tell them. If you need them to go faster, slower, a little to the left or right, tell them. If you are watching an adult film and you see something that looks like fun, let them know. You are their sex educator and the only person who can tell them how to touch you.

How to Give and Get Great Oral Sex

- Be enthusiastic. Let your lover feel your emotions through your actions. Be worshipful, ravaging, willing, playful, dominant, or submissive. Express yourself through actions.
- Make noise. This lets your lover know you are enjoying what you are doing or receiving. Even little sounds can be very encouraging. If you are giving oral sex keep in mind the fact that the noises you make actually turn your mouth into a subtle vibrator, hence the name "hummer" when referring to a great blowjob.
- Tune in to your lover. Use every sense you have to listen to your lover's body. When you feel their pelvis rising and hear breath getting deeper, those are your signals that you are doing something right. Tune in to the person giving as well. Do they look fatigued? Are they in a comfortable

position? Are they enjoying themselves? Look for even
the slightest clues.

- Ask questions. Teeth or no teeth? Should I use a toy? No
toy? Fingers inside you? No fingers? Harder? Softer?
Faster? Slower?

- You have more than a mouth, use both your hands as
well.

- Give generously. It can be fun to go down spontaneously
on your lover and ask for nothing in return.

- Be a generous receiver. Lay back and let your lover take
you sometimes with no regard for having to reciprocate
the pleasure. Let yourself be spoiled!

- Connect with your lover from time to time. Flash them a
little eye contact to show them you are there, tuned in, and
enjoying what is happening.

- Give your lover explicit, honest compliments on their
body. Find what you like and say it. "I love the way you
taste." "You have a beautiful pussy." "I love the girth of
your cock." "I love the vein that runs up the underside
of your penis." Most of us do not get enough admira-
tion when it comes to our bodies and sexuality. When
someone gives you a compliment on your body it makes
you want to hop into bed and show off what you've got!

- If you have facial hair, you may want to cover your lover's
inner thighs with a towel or sheet to protect their skin.

- Have safer sex. Use condoms and dental dams.

- Practice! Practice! Practice!

How do I get my lover to enjoy going down on me?

There can be a bunch of reasons why a person may shy away from giving or receiving oral sex. They may not like having pubic hair in their mouth. That can totally freak some people out. You might try grooming your pubic hair and see how your lover responds. Maybe they like pubic hair and you shave it?

They also may not like the taste or smell of your body or any body for that matter. If that's the case you could invite your partner to have foreplay in the shower with you. This way both of you will have a chance to use soap and water as a part of your sex play. But if you are having safer sex and using latex barriers like condoms and dental dams, your partner really should not taste your body.

Perhaps your lover does not feel confident with their technique? Maybe they do not know how to bring you to orgasm with their mouth? Maybe they were brought up to believe giving oral sex makes a person slutty or that a person's sexual anatomy is ugly and dirty? Perhaps your lover looks at giving oral sex as a submissive act and they prefer being in control? There are lots of possible explanations.

Speak with your lover about your desire for more oral sex. Keep an open mind and listen to their response. Speak in positives. Tell them why you love their mouth and how it feels for you. Let them know you wish to find a way to make oral sex enjoyable for them, too. In the end, oral sex simply may not be their cup of tea, but the only way to find out is to explore the matter with your partner.

How do you keep pubic hair from getting in your mouth while performing oral sex?

You can shave with a razor, crop down and groom your pubic hair with a beard trimmer, or you can use one hand to cover the pubic hair that gets in your way. If your partner's hair is really bothering you, let them know. But if you want them to shave their genital area, you should be prepared to shave yours, too.

HOMEWORK:

Here's a funny but very enlightening exercise to help you understand just how sexy you are. Look at your mouth in the mirror. Look at it as the sex tool that it is. Use a banana, an ice-cream cone, half a peach or mango as your object of desire and practice your techniques. If you do it in front of a mirror you can see just how sexy your mouth really is and get some good ideas of how you can use it to tease and tempt your lover!

How can I orgasm while receiving oral sex?

Not everyone orgasms while receiving oral sex. That does not mean that it does not feel great. It just means the sensation only takes that person so far before they need or want to move on to something else.

With that said, you can try engaging your mind and body in different ways to see where oral sex might take you. For example you may want to try flexing your pelvic muscles during oral sex, take deep breaths, try a new position, lose yourself in a raunchy sex fantasy, watch your lover, use your hand or your favorite sex toy in conjunction with their mouth, watch a porn film, try it with a blindfold or try it with your legs tied to the bed frame with soft rope! The possibilities are endless and the worst-case scenario is that you may not orgasm. At least you will have fun trying!

Does the person giving head feel pleasure when giving oral sex?

People feel pleasure while giving oral sex and for various reasons. Some people get pleasure out of seeing their lover enjoying themselves. Other people enjoy a feeling of power that comes with taking their lover in their mouth. They may feel dominant, as if they are taking away their lover's sense of control and demanding an orgasm from the receiver. Other people enjoy a feeling of submission from giving oral sex, as if they're serving their lover. Some people will get incredibly turned on by being the giver. For a select few, giving oral sex will even bring them to orgasm. Never underestimate the power of giving pleasure.

Is it safe to go down on your girlfriend with a menthol cough drop in your mouth?

Some women (and men) really love the feeling of menthol. If you look at the active ingredients in most of the female sexual enhancement products and in the slew of warming lubricants that have hit the market you will see menthol listed.

If she loves the feeling of menthol, then I recommend using a sugar-free cough drop because you'll want to avoid getting sugar in her vagina. Use it on her clit, nipples, or any other part, but just not inside her vaginal lips and vagina. For some women getting sugar in their vagina may throw off their natural ecology and lead to a yeast infection, especially if they have a tendency to get them anyway.

Or you could achieve the same effect by using the smallest dab of toothpaste or mouthwash. I say use a small amount because with menthol, a little goes a long way!

When you go down on a woman, do most women enjoy penetration with a tongue?

Most women want and need clit stimulation to get off, but using your tongue in her vaginal opening and on her lips might feel good. This sensation may get her excited and bring blood flow into the whole area. When in doubt, ask her if she likes it.

True Tales of Going Down On Her:

"My very first boyfriend was the best. He would not let things get too wet. I like it when the guy's tongue is more on the dry side so that you really feel what he is doing and just running his tongue around every area possible and mixing up the direction, pace, and pressure. One thing I absolutely can't stand is when the guy "slobbers" and it gets so wet down there that I feel the need to towel off. It kills it for me since I feel nothing then."

"One trick I learned is in positioning. If you have a partner that likes to be penetrated while receiving oral sex, it's awkward if you're positioned between her legs. If you position yourself beside her instead (so that you are basically perpendicular to her), you can still use your tongue on her clit, and your hand is in a much better position for fucking her at the same time."

❝ Eye contact. Everything else depends on your partner, but eye contact while giving and receiving oral sex is pretty universally hot. ❞

"If I'm getting pleasure, I like it very soft at first. I don't mind a little hard action sex sometimes, but not with my clit. Licking my clit and using a small vibrator or finger to push on the g-spot on the inside with totally makes me orgasm."

"Start slow with lots of teasing. Most women don't like it when you go straight for the clit. You have to go everywhere else on her body first and make her think you're never ever going to get to her clit. Make her beg for it. Always remember that there are other parts to the vulva besides the clit. Try sucking and licking on her inner and outer labia. When with a new partner start very slowly and softly as she may be super-sensitive and you could hurt her. Watch for cues in figuring out what she likes. Experiment. If she likes g-spot stimulation search for it, don't just assume its location. Be open to using sex toys. A cordless vibrating bullet can add a world of fun to the scene."

"My experience with oral sex varies greatly from partner to partner. Every woman I have ever been with has their own different little things that they like that sets them apart from the others. For example, one woman I was with had a very sensitive clit and couldn't take very much direct contact with it from my tongue, while other girls could not get enough. The best thing to do is work with your partner and find out all their little quirks about how they like to get oral. Communication really is the best thing you can do if you want to improve your orgasms. And just use your common sense. If you're doing something that makes them arch their back, gasp for air, and pull your hair at the same time, you're probably doing something right."

I really don't like the smell of vaginas and I heard the taste isn't very good either. Is there any kind of advice you can give me to get over my hang-up with cunnilingus?

Oral sex is an acquired taste. You have to do it a few times to understand why it tastes good! It's so much more than just the scent or the flavor in your mouth. It's the rising and the grinding of her hips in your face and noises she will make when you do it right.

If it is the smell and taste that has you hesitating, you may want to coax her into the tub or shower. Use the shower as a prelude to sex. Draw her a bath and use your hands to stimulate her while you clean her. If you're shy about talking about it, she does not even need to know your plan; let her believe your fun in the tub is simply foreplay.

Also remember that going down on someone without a latex

barrier is not safe sex. So in all honestly, unless you are in a committed relationship and have both been tested, you should be using a dental dam or nonmicrowavable plastic wrap. This protects your mouth from her vagina and her vagina from your mouth. It keeps both of you from passing possible STDs, infections, or bacteria. If you explain to her that you are using a barrier because you care about her, then you will be able to go down on her all day and never have to worry about the taste.

Does a dental dam make oral sex less pleasurable for the receiver?

Dental dams are damn sexy! A dam is a very thin, sensual square of latex. Every time I have one in my hands I dream of having a dress made entirely of dental dams! I'm not kidding. I find dental dams to be erotic.

She may be able to tell there is a barrier between your mouth and her pussy. The more you use a dental dam, the better you will become at it and less she will recognize that you are using one.

Start by using a little lube on the side of the dental dam that will be touching her pussy. This will help hold the dam in place and it will give her a sensation of wetness to go with the warmth of your mouth.

Any inconvenience or initial awkwardness you may experience while using a dam is made up for by the fact that you know you are protecting her pussy and your mouth at the same time. Using safer sex materials is a token of love. Even if you are having sex with someone you barely know, you are still loving you!

> **FACT:**
>
> In rare cases, blowing air into a woman's vaginal opening can cause an embolism (force air into her bloodstream) and it might actually kill her. If you like to play with breath and blowing air on her pussy, it's best if you breathe on her external parts, like her clit and vulva.

Is oral sex safer than vaginal sex?

Any time you make the choice to have sex you may be putting yourself at risk. One benefit of having oral sex over vaginal sex is that with oral sex there is no risk of pregnancy. Anything you can do to keep from getting pregnant before you are ready is a smart move. Here's how the risks can be weighed.

Totally Safe

Fantasies, masturbation, phone sex, computer sex, dry sex through your clothing.

Pretty Safe

- Kissing. Leaves you vulnerable to colds, flu, and hepatitis B. Try to be careful not to kiss someone who is or has recently been sick. Get a hepatitis B vaccine.
- Protected oral, vaginal, or anal sex. Leaves you vulnerable to herpes and warts (HPV) if they are outside of the area

covered by your condom or dam. If you see a lesion or open sore on your partner, avoid sex until they have seen a doctor to address the situation.

More Risky

- Hands, fingers in vagina or butt. Having any cuts or scratches on your hands leaves you vulnerable to hepatitis B, herpes, HIV, and warts (HPV). Use gloves or a condom over your fingers to protect yourself.
- Unprotected oral sex on him. Leaves you vulnerable to gonorrhea, hepatitis B, herpes, HIV, syphilis, and warts (HPV). Use a condom to protect yourself.
- Unprotected oral sex on her when she does not have her period. Leaves you vulnerable to gonorrhea, hepatitis B, herpes, HIV, syphilis, and warts (HPV). Use a dental dam or plastic wrap to protect yourself.

High Risk

- Unprotected vagina/penis sex. Leaves you vulnerable to pregnancy, chlamydia, gonorrhea, hepatitis B, herpes, HIV, and warts (HPV). Use a condom to protect yourself.
- Unprotected anal sex. Leaves you vulnerable to chlamydia, gonorrhea, hepatitis B, herpes, HIV, and (HPV). Use a condom to protect yourself.
- Unprotected oral sex on her when she has her period. Leaves you vulnerable to chlamydia, gonorrhea, hepatitis B, herpes, HIV, and warts (HPV). Use a dental dam or plastic wrap to protect yourself.

How can I keep my momentum going while giving oral sex?

It is important to recognize that not everyone will orgasm from oral sex. If you are tired you may want to ask your partner if they feel an orgasm coming on. If not, switch positions; move on to some other kind of sensation like using your hands, a sex toy, or vaginal penetration.

If you want to keep going with oral sex but you are uncomfortable, make sure you are in a position that supports your body. You and your lover can lie on your sides so you can use their thigh as a pillow to support your neck. Or you can set your lover up in a chair so you can keep your back straight. Whatever position you choose, the better your body is supported, the longer you will be able to maintain that position.

Breathe through your nose, this way your mouth can relax and not choke while trying to catch a breath. Also, let your saliva pool rather than trying to hold it in. This will also help your mouth and throat relax. Plus it make your oral fun sloppy and more animal-like!

Use your hand. Let them do most of the work while your mouth is the warm, wet subtle sensation. You can use your fingers on her clit or on his shaft. Or you can let your hands explore their vagina, butt, balls, inner thighs, etc.

Use sex toys. Explore their body with a sex toy while you go down on them. You can even try using the sex toy through your cheek or under your chin for a fun sensation.

Is there a secret to making a guy come quickly when you are getting tired of giving a blowjob?

Sometimes. It depends upon the guy. Some guys want the blowjob to be a slow buildup because they have more intense orgasms that way. But if you are exhausted and looking to get him off sooner, start by letting him know. Many guys will be able to help you inspire an orgasm just by flexing their muscles or getting conscious around the fact that it's time to orgasm.

You could try keeping your hand and mouth rhythm as consistent as possible. Most guys will orgasm from a constant pumping action.

You might incorporate perineum sensation with your blowjob. The perineum is the area between his balls and his anus and can be an extremely responsive area for some men. Not only do you find more erectile tissue from the root of his penis in this spot but, just as with the female body, all of the male pelvic muscles come together at this one area. This is the area where you should try using your fingers, tongue, and/or vibrator on him.

With his balls in your hand, inch your fingers toward his perineum. I recommend using the pads of two or three of your fingers rather than the pinpoint pressure of a single finger. Use your finger pads to create rhythmic pressure, pushing gently into his body. You'll feel the root of his penis and the tight band of pelvic muscles. Another touch you may want to try in this area is to use those same three finger pads to do a circular massage. Be aware of his response to see if you should use more pressure or less.

Some people report that stimulating their guy's perineum results in an instant orgasm because it puts pressure on the prostate through the outside of his body. Another way to put pressure on the prostate, if he's into it, is to slip a lubricated finger into his butt and do a delicate tapping motion towards his navel.

Or the two of you may decide it's a good time to flip things around, try a different sex act or position so you can continue to enjoy the experience.

Does a man prefer it if you go up and down with your tongue or around and around?

He might like both! Try each move and watch his reaction. Look for subtle signs of enjoyment like a change in breathing, hip movements, and noises he might make. Or be more direct. Try the move and ask him yes-or-no questions. "Do you like this? Faster? Slower?" Each man is different in what he likes and only he can tell you what feels good for him. You just have to find the right way to coax out his secrets!

True Tales of Going Down on Him:

"My advice? Enjoy it, make eye contact, pay attention to what works and what doesn't, be prepared to be told something doesn't feel good and be able to take it with a smile (a coy smile, a gentle lick, and "well, then, I won't do that again"). Never forget that there is more going on than just oral sex. I like to rub my breasts against the person's thighs or run a hand along their hip. I stop and kiss other places. Straddling their leg just to drip on them while performing oral sex works, too. It's one way they know you're enjoying it."

" Doesn't matter if her style or technique is a little off. . . . If she can make me think she loves what she's doing and that she's doing it because it turns her on, then that makes it a million percent better. **"**

"My boyfriend loves it when he's lying on his back and I kneel between his legs and I suck his balls and run my fingers over his perineum. After a little while, I look him in the eye, run my tongue up his shaft, and when I get to the tip, I take his whole shaft in my mouth."

"Communication really is the key to pleasing your partner in oral sex or any kind of sex. Watching and listening for signs and asking what they like. The absolute worst thing you can do is to go down on your new partner like you went down on your ex-lover and insist that your ex liked it, so they must also. Guys like lots of hand usage. You can use your hand to go up and down and twirl with your mouth, you can use your hand when your mouth gets tired, you can use your hand to tease, and you can use your other hand to play with their balls or perineum. Use lots of saliva. Flick your tongue against his perineum. And above all enjoy doing what you're doing. That can make all the difference in the world."

"I tend to go for teasing, paying attention to every part but the penis for as long as possible, then when you do get onto it taking time to move from soft kissing through to licking, then sucking, slowly getting the hands more involved. Special attention to the underside of the shaft, under the glans, frenulum, and the opening to the urethra with your tongue."

"Find something your partner likes and pay attention to even the slightest reaction, since the quietest moan can tell you if you are on the right tack or not. Also, one should not be afraid to ask, since some people might be too shy to just come out and say what they want in fear of offending a person."

"I like to incorporate some variation. Switch from sucking hard to lightly, switch to licking and flick my tongue along the tip. I also keep my hands involved and either play with the balls or rub the shaft. I like to lightly nibble on the balls and run my teeth along the shaft and depending on his mood I might be a bit rougher with my teeth."

"I wander off with my mouth and kinda just leave him 'hanging' while I will kiss him everywhere but there. I'll kiss and lick his stomach, his chest and ears, then work my way down, past his groin and all the way down his leg and toes and then work my way up and just build the anticipation."

"Eye contact is always a big plus. I also like it when he strokes my face in the process or runs his fingers through my hair."

"I think the main thing is that a lot of men I have talked to have said how many women pay too much attention to the penis and not nearly enough to the balls. When starting off I have my hand around the base of the penis with fingers around the balls (trying to get them around far enough to put some pressure behind/under the balls). Kiss them, lick them, stick them in your mouth, and try to feel them as much as possible with your spare hand."

What is the best way to deep-throat his penis or at least take as much as possible without gagging?

Your gag reflex is a really, really important muscle. It keeps you from choking on food and dying. By nature some people are born with a tight gag reflex while others have a very loose one. You may or may not be able to learn to relax your gag reflex, depending upon how your body is built and how big your partner's penis may be.

For most people the gag reflex is located about three inches behind the teeth. The average erect penis is about five to six inches. If you are a person with a naturally relaxed gag reflex, you may be able to slip those inches deeper into your throat. But there a lot of people who have tighter gag reflexes. Some people are so sensitive in this area that they cannot even swallow pills without crushing them.

With that said, a great deal of one's ability to deep-throat or not deep-throat has to do with your natural ability. If you want to see if you can take more length with your mouth, you can try breathing through your nose and consciously trying to relax your throat muscles. But even doing this may be difficult, with the stress of having him thrusting in and out of your mouth. Whatever you do, be gentle

> **FACT:**
>
> According to sexologist Alfred Kinsey, chimpanzees can suck themselves off and do so often, but only two or three out of a thousand men can suck themselves off.

and kind to your throat. What you cannot take with your mouth can always be swallowed up by a nice wet hand job at the base of his penis while your mouth works the head.

If you orgasm by way of oral sex is it acceptable to cum inside your girlfriend's mouth? Should you warn her?

You should talk to her about what her preference is before she ever puts her mouth on your penis. It is much easier to get what you want and to give her what she wants if you ask.

Beyond that, you should not ejaculate in her mouth. If you want to cum while in her mouth, you should wear a condom and let the condom catch your cum. This is great for a number of reasons. You protect your penis from her mouth. You protect her mouth from your penis. The best part of having a latex barrier is that you can enjoy the blowjob and not have to hesitate or worry about how and when to ejaculate.

Should one spit or swallow during oral sex?

Neither. If you're practicing safer sex you should let him have his explosive orgasm outside of your body or in a condom. Swallowing or holding his ejaculate in your mouth can also be unsafe.

People have this idea that oral sex is safer than vaginal or anal sex. It's not true. If you respect yourself and your partner, don't ask them to have unsafe oral sex with you. And please don't ask them to swallow. Use condoms for oral sex. Pick up some of the super-delicious, unlubricated Lifestyles Kiss of Mint condoms or any other flavored condom.

You may be wondering how this could be fun or you may be cursing me for telling you like it is, but I honestly care about you. I want you to have healthy parts and I want you to have fun.

To make this tough-love lesson in safer oral sex a little easier to swallow (so to speak!), try putting a couple drops of lube inside the condom before you roll it down on his penis. This will give him some wetness to go with the warmth of your mouth and provide more pleasurable friction.

If he gives you a little warning that he is about to cum, happily ask him where he wants it. It can be totally hot for him to ejaculate on your breasts or on your ass. Have fun with the whole thing and make his orgasm a celebration! Doing it this way is so much more fun than the risks of unsafe oral sex or trying to swallow only to make that sour face that some people make when they taste cum. That face is not so sexy!

Is there something a man can do to make his cum sweeter and less bitter?

The better your diet and the more hydrated you are, the better you will taste. For example you could cut out junk food, cigarettes, and alcohol and you would taste better. Even your mouth will taste better.

Some people say if you increase the amount of natural fructose in your diet that you will taste better. Fructose can be found in most noncitrus fruits like peaches, pears, bananas, and berries. There could be some truth to this, considering that fructose is a naturally occurring ingredient in the composition of semen.

The bad news is that semen has other ingredients that tend to outshine the sweet fructose, like ammonia. Which is why it is healthy and normal for a guy's ejaculate to smell and taste a little like a cleaning product.

But if you are having safer oral sex you should be using condoms for oral sex and not tasting his ejaculate at all.

Chemical Composition of Ejaculate

Ammonia
Ascorbic acid
Ash
Calcium
Carbon dioxide
Chloride
Cholesterol
Citric acid
Copper
Creatine
Ergothionine
Fructose
Glutathione

Glycerylphosphoryl-choline

Inositol

Lactic acid

Lipid

Magnesium

Nitrogen, nonprotean

Phosphorus (acid soluble)

Phosphorylcholine

Potassium

Pyruvic Acid

Sodium

Sorbitol

Vitamin B_{12}

Sulfur

Uric acid

Zinc

Does licking a man's balls have any benefit?

Absolutely. Some guys love the way it feels when you use your mouth on his balls. In Chapter 9 I explained how an individual's gender is determined in the womb. We all start out with the same basic form. Our pelvic skin can grow into labia lips or scrotum. If you are a female, use this fact as your guide for understanding how the skin on his balls may react to touch—very similar to the skin of your vaginal lips. Don't hesitate to explore this area of his body. Touch him the ways you like to have your lips touched and see how he responds.

18.

Intercourse: The Ins & Outs

How often do women orgasm during penetrative sex with their partner?

The truth is that it is normal *not* to orgasm during intercourse, or to orgasm during penetration only, so long as she has some kind of clitoral stimulation as well. This does not mean that vaginal penetration does not feel good for women. It means you have to amplify that sensation by touching her clit and/or encouraging her to touch herself. Many women report that nothing compares to having both clitoral and vaginal stimulation simultaneously.

What sexual position optimizes clitoral stimulation?

Any position that makes it possible for you to rub as much of her vulva as possible during penetration may be able to take her there. You can do this in the missionary position (her on the bottom and

> ## FACT:
>
> Of the three thousand women who participated in the 1976 nationwide study of female sexuality entitled *The Hite Report*, only 26 percent experienced orgasm from intercourse on a regular basis. With deeper inquiry, researchers found that only two out of every ten women could experience orgasms without clitoral stimulation. Most women report that they need hands, vibrators, or oral sex to get off.

you on top) if her legs are spread wide and you make sure your pubic bone and lower belly are making contact with as much of her vulva and pubic mound as possible. With each thrust you will be rubbing vulva and at least causing a tugging sensation on her clit. This is even easier if you have a bit of a belly. (Beer bellies can be especially good at this position. Finally, a legitimate excuse to drink beer!)

When in doubt, just use your fingers on her clit, reach down and around or whatever you need to do. If you know that's what it takes to get her off, then go for it!

Another great way to achieve clit-induced orgasms during penetrative play is with sex toys. You could use one of the many vibrating cock rings. Your cock or dildo goes through the ring. The ring has a vibrating attachment that curves over her pubic bone and stimulates her clit. Or you can take a strong vibrator, like the Hitachi Magic Wand, put it down on the bed and have intercourse from behind (doggy-style) with her pelvis pressed down onto the vibrator.

What is the secret of women who orgasm from penetration alone?

You may or may not be able to orgasm during penetration, but why not try? Do whatever you can to strengthen your pelvic muscles (like the exercises outlined in Chapter 6) and flex them during penetrative play. As I have said, the stronger your pelvic muscles are, the stronger your orgasms will be.

How can I learn to stay present and have an orgasm with a partner?

As humans we have an amazing ability to survive whatever life may throw at us. In order to cope we may zone out, drain our brain, go numb. Or we watch movies, television, read, sleep, or get drunk. We disappear in some intangible way.

Many of us, myself included, survive by retreating into ourselves. This coping mechanism can help us get by day to day, especially if we have survived sexual, physical, or emotional abuse in our lives. But at some point we realize this behavior can be an obstacle in our relationships and especially in our sex lives.

To have hot, satisfying, mind-blowing, connected sex you must be present and aware. To do that you need to be engaged with your mind, body, and breathing and tuned in with yourself and your lover as well. Learning to be present can be frustrating and scary sometimes, if tuning out has been a survival skill for you.

Take little steps. Start by turning off the television or whatever distractions provide an escape from your thoughts, body, and self. Ride a bike, do yoga, stretch, learn martial arts, walk your dog, take a shower, get a massage, or masturbate. Take deep breaths, tune in, and listen to your body. Do one thing every day just for your physical self. Do it for the rest of your life.

When you are having sex with your partner, start by taking little steps as well. With each encounter try to incorporate the following, one by one, as you are ready:

- Breathe and listen to your breath before, during, and after sex play.
- Flex your pelvis muscles rhythmically as you breathe.
- Watch for subtle responses in your lover's body, such as their breath and movements.
- Share a little eye contact with your partner.
- If you feel yourself "checking out" during sex, gently guide yourself back into the moment by breathing and paying attention to your breath. Try not to get too frustrated with yourself if you find this process to be difficult.

As you grow and change, try to find fun ways to interact and communicate with your partner. For example, you could make an effort to eat breakfast together, go on walks, dance, sleep in a tent on the lawn for no reason, read erotica to each other, play Scrabble with extra letters and only sexy words, or cook foods the two of you find to be erotic.

All of these seemingly unrelated acts really do add up to living more truly in your skin and more orgasms for both of you.

> ### MYTH:
>
> While the idea of simultaneous orgasms (both partners cli-
> maxing at the same time) may be romantic when depicted in a
> film or novel, the reality is that simultaneous orgasms seldom
> happen. Generally women take longer than men and may want
> more than one orgasm. The best you can do is try to make
> sure everyone who wants an orgasm gets one. Rather than
> having goal-oriented sex, take the pressure off yourself and
> your lover and simply seek to enjoy the journey.

What is the average time for sex?

According to a survey conducted by Harris Interactive the average
sexual encounter lasts fifteen to thirty minutes. The condom company Durex did a study that proved most Americans do it at 10:34
in the evening, and *Esquire* magazine reported the most common
frequency seems to be two to three times per week.

But average is boring. Be yourself. Check in with your partner to
find out if they are happy. Ask them, "Are we having sex often
enough? Are you getting what you want?" Shake it up. Add some
spontaneity to your play. Have sex outside of your bedroom. If you
normally have sex at night, try doing it in the morning or afternoon.
Try a new position or sex toy. Try not to compare yourself to statistics. They can be interesting, but in reality statistics can vary greatly
depending upon the gender, orientation, age, race, religion, culture,
and class of the people polled. Don't compare yourself to anyone or

anything. Find your pleasure where you feel most happy and work to keep your partner(s) happy, too.

What is the most innovative new sexual position?

Innovative? I don't think there are too many positions that have not already been discovered and documented over the centuries. But that does not mean some of these positions could not be innovative and new to you!

Go to a bookstore that carries sex books and you will find there are oodles of illustrated books dedicated to exploring sex positions. You may want to check out *Position of the Day: Sex Every Day in Every Way*, by the folks at nerve.com. Books like this one can be inspiring, fun, and even funny. You may find some things you want to try and will definitely find some acrobatic positions; a few of them require you to be a circus contortionist to pull them off!

In truth, the best sex positions are the ones that are comfortable for your body and your lover's body. You want to support your back and neck. You don't want your arms to have to hold your body weight for extended periods of time. You want your knees to lie on something soft.

I recommend looking at the furniture in your house to see which innovative positions you can enjoy over the back of your couch, over the arm of a padded chair, on your carpeted steps, on your countertops, or on various chairs you may own. In bed, pull pillows into place to raise your hips or support your head. Look at your lover. Are they straining in any way? Are their knees on a safe surface? Care for them.

You'll also find the more you work out and strengthen the muscles in every area of your body, the more sexual positions you will be able to achieve comfortably. Great positions are the ones we can maintain for at least some period of time.

— · — · —

True Tales of Great Positions:

"I would have to say missionary, with my hips raised on something (stack of pillows). Given the height difference between my husband and me this is the best position for him to be comfortable and for my g-spot to be hit during intercourse. As long as we have had a lot of foreplay beforehand and my body is completely warmed up, I will usually orgasm in this position."

—·—·—·—·—·—·—·—·—·—·—·—·—·—·—·—·—

❝ Nothin' says lovin' like sitting on the bathroom sink (butt on the ledge) with my partner penetrating me while standing next to the aforementioned sink. Just sitting up a bit (versus lying down for missionary) helps me find my g-spot faster! Countertops work well, too, but I always feel a little weird having lovin' in the kitchen and then cooking in it. It's hard to lay down the contents of a bologna sandwich while thinking, 'My ass was here'.**❞**

—·—·—·—·—·—·—·—·—·—·—·—·—·—·—·—·—

"Lots of positions are nifty; still it's the missionary position I appreciate. If you can still call it 'missionary' when one of the parties is wearing a strap-on cock. There's still something infinitely magical about looking your partner in the eye when you're face-to-face."

"I find different positions are more fun with different partners. With one ex of mine, I used to lie facedown on the mattress with my legs closed and he'd fuck me with his legs around mine. It was really really good. Then I tried it with my husband, and, well, it was utterly unsatisfying. These days, I tend to prefer doggy-style, though I often start with me on top, and I've lately found a love of reverse cowgirl. Still, those are often the starter positions, and then finishing doggy-style."

"Missionary, because I am lazy! But doggy-style is also good, since it's the easiest way to use my Magic Wand (which is the only way I can come from penetrative sex)."

"I have to admit to favoring doggy-style, and fortunately my wife does, too. But we switch up all the time during sex and change positions. It usually ends up doggy-style at the finish line, but in between there are position changes."

What is the best sex position for a woman to achieve an orgasm?

The smaller percentage of women who can have an orgasm from penetration alone report that being on top as their most orgasmic position. Ideally, she is lying on top of him, chest-to-chest and face-to-face. She will move her body forward and back, rather than up and down.

I prefer to be on top but it seems guys prefer other positions. Any suggestions for how to make both of us happy?

This straddling position, with you face-to-face and chest-to-chest on top of him, with a back-and-forth thrusting method is usually not as comfortable for him, and I have had conversations with lots of women who have encountered some conflict with their partner while in this position.

Guys generally like it if their partner sits straight up and does an up and down stroke. But many women report this straight-up position is not as comfortable because this allows deeper penetration and he ends up bumping her cervix (a sensitive spot for some women).

I recommend that whenever possible each partner compromise a little. She should let him see her hop up and down some. She can use her thigh muscles to hold herself up and not let the strokes go too deep. When doing this I want you to understand one very important thing: every woman, no matter how big or small her breasts may be, looks great in this position. Our tits look fantastic from the underside view. Most women would not know this of course because we cannot see our own breasts from that perspective. But you look hot! I promise you. You could take advantage of your own hotness by flipping your hair around and showing off!

Whenever possible, guys should allow their female partner to lean over and claim her orgasm. Women know this position may not be as comfortable for men, but guys should be willing to accommodate their female partners. Lie back and enjoy the experience of having her have her way with you!

What is a man's favorite sexual position?

When I did a poll on my Web site, the more than two hundred men who responded all had different preferences. The favorite position really depends upon the man. His answer can also vary depending upon where he is having sex, how able or disabled his body may be, who he is having sex with, and a multitude of other variables. Ask your guy. If a little time passes, ask him again and see if he has something new in mind!

I like to have sex "doggy-style" more often than I do at the moment because my wife complains that it is painful. Is that common?

Yes. Doggy-style makes it possible for you to achieve deeper penetration. (Unless she has a big butt like J. Lo and me!) When you go deeper you can bump her cervix with each stroke. Some women enjoy this sensation and others, like your wife, find it to be painful.

Try having her push her legs out behind her and ease her down onto her tummy a little. Prop her up with pillows if it makes the position more comfortable for her. This allows her thighs to block the depth of your stroke. If she is still in pain or finds this position uncomfortable, have her go all the way down on her tummy so she is lying flat on the bed. This way her butt and thighs will create a buffer for her vagina. Use plenty of lube and you may achieve an intense sensation as you move in and out of the lushness of her thighs and butt as you penetrate her vaginally.

Every time we have sex doggy-style we have all this air build up and my pussy makes funny sounds. How can we do this position without that happening?

Ah, the dreaded pussy whoopee cushion! It happens to almost everyone sooner or later. The cause of this sound is not in your pussy, but in your partner's stroke. With the out stroke, they quickly exit your pussy, allowing air to enter. So when they plunge in next they force the air deeper into your pussy or right back out again, making a farting noise at the same time. Or the air can be held, deeper inside your body and exit anytime after your sex play is over.

This noise can be hilarious to some people or humiliating for others. If your body does this and the sound embarrasses you, please know it's normal. And now you know you can blame it on your partner as well!

To avoid having this happen, try to coach your partner into doing shorter strokes so that he does not pull so far away from and out of your body. If you are in a position where you can wrap you legs around him or hold him close with your arms, then that might help. For some wild buckaroos you may need both your arms and your legs!

Sometimes during sex my partner cannot stay inside me. He slips out. How can I help?

The first thing I want you to look at is the way his erection hangs. Some guys when erect will point up toward their own navel, other guys will point straight out, and some guys will point down. At the same time a woman's vagina will gently curve toward her navel. Your goal is to get your vaginal curve to go the same direction as the curve of his erection. (I always say, look at how he is hung and figure out how you wanna hop on that thing!) You want to arrange for a position where his penis is pointing toward your navel. If he points straight or toward his navel, then you might try missionary position. If he points straight out or down then you might try doggy-style.

Also look at the length of his penis and the length of his strokes. If his penis is short, it's more difficult for him to stay in as he thrusts in and out of you. No matter what his size, you want to shorten his strokes so that he does not pull so far away from and out of your body. If you are in a position where you can wrap your legs around him or hold him close with your arms, that might help, too.

Sometimes guys who are less experienced or younger are very exuberant in how they thrust and are simply sloppy. If this is your guy you may need to ask him to slow down a bit so that you can have fun, too.

What is the best way to do double penetration?

Double penetration, for anyone who does not know, means having something in her pussy and her butt at the same time. It's a big fantasy for some women, while many others are actually making it happen! Use your imagination and you can find many ways to enjoy double penetration.

Couples can try inserting his penis in her vagina while using a sex toy in her butt, or inserting his penis in her butt while using a sex toy in her vagina. You will also find lots of inventive sex toys that are made exclusively for double penetration. These toys may look unusual at first but can deliver some amazing orgasms. Another method is taking two male partners at once—one inside her pussy, with the second guy inside her butt. Not always an easy thing to arrange or experience while in a committed relationship, so this may require some negotiation and research to find an appropriate partner.

What happens after I have an orgasm and it gets dry but the guy is not ready to cum and needs to keep going?

Use lube! It's a great way to care for your body and have longer bouts of intercourse.

If your body is still not able to keep going, then you may try reaching down between your legs and wrapping your hand around the base of his penis. This way the length of his strokes that are in your body will be shorter, cutting down on friction, and you can use your hand to deliver more sensation to him.

How can you have sex in the water without getting water up your vagina and losing lubrication?

If you are submerged in water, like in a pool or hot tub, he should keep his strokes short and stay closer to your body. He should be able to block most of the water with his body as long as he does not pull all the way out. Another option is to have fun with your hands and hold off with the penetration until after you are out of the water.

In recent years we have seen the advent of silicon-based lubricants. They work really well with water because they are not water based. Water will not rinse this lube away, which makes it ideal for tub, shower, or any kind of wet play. Silicone-based lubes are more expensive but well worth the price. A little bit goes a long way.

You may have heard safer sex advocates stressing that you should only use water-based lube with condoms or other latex barriers, but silicone is another type of lube that is safe to use with latex.

Is it safe for a guy to spit on himself to lube up before intercourse? Will the germs in his saliva cause a problem in the vagina?

Using spit as a lubricant may feel good to some people but it is not the safest thing to do. You could be exposed to germs or bacteria, which in rare cases can cause vaginal or urinary infections.

If your vagina burns after sex (even after peeing), what can help?

This kind of trouble can totally ruin your sexual enjoyment! But there is hope. I would like to start by reaffirming that peeing after sex is an excellent thing to do. It flushes out your urethra and can help prevent urinary tract infections. Keep doing that.

If you have symptoms that resemble yeast infections, burning sensations, urinary tract infections, redness or swelling for extended periods of time, and/or numbness, you should see your doctor right away. Ask to be tested for bacterial, viral, and sexually transmitted infections. Ask specifically for all three of those categories. You may need medical treatment. Try not to be shy when asking for these tests. Doctors perform them everyday and a good doctor will make no judgment of you other than that you are a smart woman who is looking to care for her body. (If you don't have a good doctor, check out *"How to Find a Sex-Positive Doctor"* in Chapter 12.)

Once you have ruled out infection, do some research of your own.

First, some women are allergic to or get inflammation from perfumes, deodorants, dye (like they have in colorful toilet paper), bubble bath, alcohol, lotions, and oils. (A woman may have similar problems if she has obsessive hygiene habits or douches.) Assess whether or not you have been using any personal products that may be irritating your body.

Next, if you are not using lubricant you should try using some. You could be suffering from slight friction burn that intercourse may cause.

If you are using lubricant, try experimenting with different brands. You could be having an allergic reaction to an ingredient in your lube. Many of the best sex toy shops will carry little sample containers of various lubes. (I have listed the toy shops that carry the best products in the Resources section at the back of the book.) Try as many lubes as you can and see if one of them leaves you feeling better after sex. If you save the packages, you may also be able to compare the ingredients list and figure out what you are reacting to. I know I prefer lubricants without alcohol in them. If they do have alcohol I feel a burning sensation and totally feel like I am having an allergic reaction. Other women can use lubes with alcohol and have no problem. This is why you need to experiment for yourself.

The next thing you might consider is the kind of condom you are using. A few people are allergic to latex. You might try using a non-latex condom like Avanti-brand condoms. They will still protect you from pregnancy and sexually transmitted disease but are not made of latex.

To add more to the mix, if you are using spermicide, try discontinuing its use. Many condoms have spermicide on them, contraceptive sponges also contain spermicide, and it may be in the jelly you are using with your diaphragm. Spermicide was once believed to offer protection against HIV and other sexually transmitted diseases. That's not true. Lots of women have reactions to the stuff that is actually putting women in more danger. When exposed to spermicide, women who are allergic to it will develop microscopic sores that leave them more vulnerable to infection of every kind, including sexually transmitted diseases. Frequently spermicide is listed as "Nonoxynol-9" on the package. You can buy condoms that have no spermicide or buy nonlubricated condoms. If you are allergic to spermicide and stop using the product that contains it you will see a change instantly.

It sounds a little grueling, but with some patience and determination you can resolve this. And you'll be so happy when you do!

19.

Butt Sex:
Bottoms Up

My best friend loves receiving anal sex and says it feels good. I am afraid it would hurt. Does anal sex actually feel good?

Yes. It feels good for many people but not everyone. The reasons some people find pleasure in this area of their body can be because there are lots of very sensitive nerves ending in the anus and strong muscles that respond well to the kind of pressure and circulation that occurs with anal play. Some women also report feeling pressure on their g-spot during anal play and guys feel pressure on their prostate.

The first step to having pleasurable anal sex is desire. If you don't want to have anal sex (or an kind of sex) you should not do it. This is especially true for anal sex because you need to be able to relax your sphincter muscles in order to receive anything in your butt.

Having anal sex simply to please your partner is usually not a good idea. You need to want to do it for your own sense of pleasure as well.

Do you have any tips for a person who is having anal sex for the first time?

Many people report that it is easier to explore anal possibilities alone the first few times. It helps alleviate any fears one might have about cleanliness or pain.

If you decide to play alone or with a partner you will need to get supplies: *lubrication, latex gloves, condoms,* and possibly some *anal sex toys* in various sizes. You need the lube because your butt has no source of natural lubrication. You can use the gloves and condoms to cover your fingers and toys. This keeps everything clean and makes for easy cleanup.

Start by getting yourself aroused in whatever manner turns you on the most, be it oral sex, hands, nipples. Think of this as waking up the whole neighborhood rather than just ringing the doorbell! The more excited you get overall, the more relaxed you will be and the better anal sex will feel. Then lube up your fingers and gently massage your perineum and anus area.

It's easier than you might imagine to slip your own finger into you anus. Instead of trying to stick your finger right in, lay the pad of your finger on one side of the circles of muscle that makes up the anus and press just that one side of the anus open. The anus will open right up to your finger. If you try to poke your finger or toy straight in, the muscles will tighten up and make entry more difficult.

If you are the person receiving penetration you can also try to bear down and push out a little as entry begins.

Take your time. Go slow. Touch your partner's genitals as you play. If you are the person giving anal sex to your partner, listen and watch their response to see if they are enjoying the play. Ask the receiver yes-or-no questions so they can easily communicate what they are feeling. With each session work up to using items of bigger size, but warm up your partner with something smaller if that is what they need to get started.

— : — · —

5 Things You Need to Have Great Anal Sex

1) Desire. If you or your partner does not want to have anal sex, don't do it. The person receiving needs to be able to relax. If they are being pressured or coerced into doing a sex act that they are not comfortable with (for any reason), then it will not feel good.

2) Lube. The butt is not self-lubricating. Use lube every time you use anything (fingers, toys, penis) on or in your partner's anus. A condom alone does not have enough lubrication on it to make anal play comfortable for the receiver.

3) Safer sex supplies. Cover anything you use for anal play with a condom or gloves. If you want to pull out and go back to vaginal play, change your condom and/or glove. If possible, wash your hands, toys, and penis as well.

4) Communication. Listen and communicate with all of your senses. If you are receiving anal play, you need to tell your partner what feels good and what does not. Tell them exactly what you need, use words like "slower," "more shallow," "deeper," "hold still for a moment." These words are actually sexy in the heat of the moment and get you what you want. If you are giving anal play you need to tune in to your lover's reactions, verbal and otherwise, and respond accordingly.

5) Relaxation. The sphincter is a strong set of muscles. They need to be relaxed to be able to receive anal sex. It also helps if the person receiving is warmed up with a massage or various kinds of sex play before you go straight for anal play. Breathing is one of the most effective ways to relax your muscles. During anal play be sure to take deep breaths. If you are giving anal play, listen to your lover's breath. If they are holding their breath, encourage them to breathe for you.

Do women actually orgasm from anal sex?

Yes. Some women report having earthshaking orgasms from anal sex alone, while many other women need clit stimulation in conjunction with anal sex. In my years of researching and teaching I have even found a few women who can orgasm only from anal sex.

An orgasm is a series of contractions in your pelvic muscles. The sphincter muscles are an interwoven part of the pelvic muscles. Whether she has an orgasm that is inspired by way of her clit, g-spot, or flexing her muscles, her sphincter muscles always contract along with all of her other pelvic muscles. It only makes sense that an act that requires any part of this muscle group to flex and experience more circulation could cause the whole muscle group to become excited.

In order to experience that kind of circulation in the anal pelvic muscles, a person must be relaxed enough to comfortably receive anal sex and to allow blood circulation throughout these muscles.

True Tales of Anal Pleasure (Or Not):

"If you are giving anal sex just be sure to use *lots* of foreplay before engaging in anal sex. Use your tongue and fingers and make sure everything is plenty slippery and relaxed before your cock goes in. And make sure the woman is comfortable with it, and be prepared to stop if she says she wants to stop and don't give her any grief about it."

"I can sometimes orgasm from anal sex, but I usually require additional stimulation on my cock or balls. It's not painful, although there can be some discomfort involved. The messiest part of anal sex for me is the lubrication—and I really recommend *not* skipping this part! Relax and take your time. When giving anal, in addition to inserting my cock or fingers, I really enjoy giving analingus. This is actually a good way to start out anal play as it relaxes the recipient."

"I love anal sex! I do not give, but happily receive and I almost always orgasm from anal sex. I used to be scared of the whole idea but that was before I'd ever experienced it. I find it's only painful when the giver doesn't quite know what they're doing or isn't as patient as they should be. The best way to have good anal sex is by talking to your partner. Tell them what feels good and what doesn't. Practice muscle control. Relax. I can't stress that enough."

"I think I enjoy the thought/the naughtiness more than the actual act. I always feel a bit butterfly-ish just beforehand. Don't be afraid to try it, but don't be afraid to back out, either. The first time I had anal sex it was more uncomfortable. The next time, I knew what to expect and it was a lot more enjoyable. I also found my favorite position is me on my back with him standing against the bed leaning in, my legs over his shoulders. I guess it's a bit more romantic. And you get the eye contact so you can gauge how the other person is doing."

"I had a girlfriend who used vibrating anal beads on me and another former girlfriend who was really into fingering my ass. I really enjoyed that. I think a lot of men would like the sensations that come with being on the receiving end of anal play but they feel as if it puts their sexual orientation into question. I would like to stress to these 'dudes' that there is nothing gay about having nerve endings stimulated and feeling awesome!"

"I have a feeling I would love it if I could get to it. Both times

I've done it were bad experiences, as neither of us really knew what we were doing and we didn't take things slowly enough. Both times it started off feeling really good, but then hurt really badly. Needless to say this has made it difficult for me to relax fully, but luckily my current boyfriend has a lot of patience. Way more than I have, really. I haven't tried giving anal sex, but I do fantasize about it."

"Sometimes I love it. Sometimes I psych myself out and can't relax. Or my partner goes too fast and then it really does hurt. Right now I think I almost like it better than vaginal sex, but maybe that's because I've been having more happy experiences with it. I've learned that, for me, being super relaxed (like, lying down on my stomach), lube, and my Magic Wand on my clit are what it takes for it to feel really good."

"I defiantly orgasm from anal sex, but when he gives me anal it's been coupled with a reach around or some type of stimulation of my cock. I am not sure what actually sparked my orgasm. I find it's not as messy as I had thought it might be. And my only fears are centered around the possible transmission of disease which can be protected against. I recommend going slow (especially if you are new to anal), lots of lube, communicate, push toward g-spot or prostate for more pleasure."

"My brain is often more into it than my ass is. I can orgasm from anal if combined with clitoral and/or vaginal stimulation, and usually it's pretty good. Sometimes it's too intense or becomes painful and I have to stop before I get off. My advice? Gloves are clean and make fingers feel smoother, but damn, cut your nails anyhow! It's often easier to penetrate yourself before allowing someone else to penetrate you. If you're the tender or tentative type, try your own gloved and lubed finger up your ass first, and maybe a butt plug or some anal beads. Rather than having someone shove a cock or cock-like thing in your ass, take control and carefully lower yourself onto it, as slowly as you like. And yeah, communicate."

" I've read so much about it and I feel I am ready to try with my boyfriend. I used to have a different outlook on it, but I progressed. I started out thinking, 'In *there*? No *way!*,' then changed to 'Well maybe when I get married or something I'll try it' to 'OK, it looks like it would be pretty good and fantasizing about it really turns me on.' I am not sure when I will be entirely ready to try it but I'm glad I've read so much on it and I am well aware of how to go about it all. **"**

"I love receiving and giving! I prefer a slender, slightly pointed cock or dildo—nothing too big or too small. It's better when I'm worked up to craving it—like getting a rim job and finger play beforehand. I find that it's most comfortable when lying side-by-side (spooning). Giving also has its own pleasures, though I've only given to men (while in the case of receiving, I've gotten it from both women and men)—I find it difficult to give while wearing a harness and dildo, because I cannot control action as much, so I generally just hold the dildo and go to town (or just use my fingers—in *gloves* of course!) As for it being messy, I've never had too much of a problem. I mean, I don't ever have anal sex when I'm feeling like I need to poo, so my bowels are generally clear. Anal sex is just one of those things that I either really want or can't have at all—it's really never in between."

What are some ways to relax before anal sex?

Try it after you have had a massage or taken a bath. Many people say that they are more relaxed and ready if they first have other types of sex play. Some people like to use a vibrator on their perineum or external area as a way to warm up. As your anal play begins you might try consciously relaxing these muscles. Take deep breaths.

If you are having a stressful day, you may find anal sex is not comfortable for you. Be kind to your body and save it for another day.

What is the difference between an anal orgasm and a clitoral or vaginal orgasm?

All orgasms are defined as being *a series of muscular contractions* but there are a number different ways you can set off these contractions. The most common way a female can reach orgasm is through stimulating her clit. Other women will be inspired to orgasm by having her g-spot stimulated. And other women still will have orgasms sparked by consciously or unconsciously engaging and flexing their pelvic muscles.

The anal muscles are part of her pelvic muscles. Stimulating these muscles can pull enough blood and oxygen into her pelvis to inspire an orgasm. Orgasms driven by pumping her muscles or through anal sex (if she likes it) may feel more deep and drawn out than a clitoral orgasm. Combining clit stimulation with anal play can be the most explosive. But of course every woman is unique. How the orgasms feel for any woman is relevant to her body alone.

A Whole New World

When I was in my early twenties I had a boyfriend who was obsessed with the idea of having anal sex. He nagged me about it like a child, "Can we have anal sex? When are you going let me have anal sex with you? How 'bout anal sex?"

Nagging and coercing another into some kind of sex act they are not into has to be one of the least sexy things a person can do. Besides, what was with his urgent curiosity about anal sex?

I was an anal virgin, and my response to him was very clear, "My ass is an exit only. There is no way you are going in my ass." And I meant it.

After being with him for a number of years, learning to trust him, and growing more secure with my own body, I found myself coming back to the idea of anal sex. I don't know if I wanted to surprise him or please him, but one day I said, "I'll tell you what, I'll let you put your finger in my butt if I can put my finger in your butt, too."

This seemed only fair. It's not like women's butt holes are more pliable than guys'. I figured we could explore the whole idea together.

Suddenly the tables were turned.

"No way! My ass is an exit only!" was his response.

He wasn't going to let me anywhere near his butt. Which was fine with me. I was off the hook! No pressure for me to give it up to him. He stopped pressuring me for anal sex and eventually we broke up. (It wasn't the anal sex thing! We were just not meant to be.)

A few years later I was talking on the phone with my friend Tonya. She is a beautiful, sex-positive, and open-minded person. We blabber on about sex at every opportunity.

In this particular conversation anal sex came up. She asked me if I had ever had it. I said no. She exclaimed, "What? Oh my god! There's a whole new world waiting for you up your ass! You've got to get in there!"

We both laughed like crazy and the conversation moved on to another topic. But Tonya's exuberant response to my inexperience with anal sex stayed with me. Suddenly I had interest in the idea—and this time for real.

I ended up buying toys and lube and experimenting on my own body. Eventually I tried it with a partner, too, and found there was indeed a whole new world waiting for me up my ass! It's different than my vaginal world. Vaginal sex is an ordinary thing for me. My anal world on the other hand is place I go on holidays. My anal sex orgasms have been intense, leaving me with feelings of vulnerability that totally surprised me. It's too intense for me to go there with every bout of sex, but every now and then it's fun to visit!

Looking back I realize that I had to hear about the pleasures of anal sex from someone who was *not* trying to have anal sex with me before I could ever believe it was true. Prior to my conversation with Tonya I always felt like the guy was trying to get something from me instead of trying to give something to me.

So in case you have never had anal sex and never heard from an honest friend that there really is pleasure in it, I would like to be that friend. I promise you, there is a whole new world waiting for you up your ass!

Can anal sex feel as good for women as it does for men?

It is difficult to compare female sexual response with male sexual response. Women find their pleasure in anal play through muscular response and a feeling of internal fullness and pressure. Men have all that—plus a prostate. The prostate is the gland that creates a huge portion of his ejaculatory fluid. It is a couple of inches inside his rectum, toward his navel. If you were to use a finger and massage as if you were trying to stroke his belly button from the inside, some guys will orgasm immediately. A toy or a penis will put lots of pressure on the prostate and cause more stimulation.

Some women have wild, explosive reactions while others find anal sex to be painful and difficult. Some guys have their best orgasms by way of anal sex while other guys find no interest in it. Sensation is always relative to the individual.

FACT:

When America's founding fathers were plotting early American government they carried over a lot of British laws, including an antiquated law declaring anal sex, or *sodomy,* illegal. In the United States these laws have been used to limit individuals right to privacy in the bedroom and to prosecute gay individuals in particular. Since the late twentieth century, activist groups and gay organizations have been working with some success to repeal existing sodomy laws. Despite this, anal sex between consenting adults is still illegal in Alabama, Florida, Idaho, Kansas, Louisiana, Mississippi, Missouri, North Carolina, Missouri, South Carolina, Utah, and Virginia.

Is it safe for pregnant women to have anal sex?

The only person who can answer this question is your doctor. A woman may be able to have the full menu of sex play options available to her during pregnancy while others may be limited in the kind of movements their doctor will allow. If you are pregnant I highly recommend picking up a copy of *Sexy Mamas: Keeping Your Sex Life Alive While Raising Kids,* by Cathy Winks and Anne Semans. They address not only sex during pregnancy but also how to maintain your sexual identity as you become parents and how to raise sex-positive kids.

Why are guys so obsessed with anal sex?

Some guys love to give it while others love to get it. Or both! Or neither. It really depends upon the guy. I did do a poll on my Web site just to get a broader idea of why a guy might be obsessed with anal sex. I found that guys who have never had anal sex are the most fixated. Once they have experienced it a few times they usually cool out. The next most common responses included,

1) "Try something different. A different sensation from the vagina. A tight ring of muscle."
2) "Control exchange. A feeling of submission or domination."
3) "Sheer naughtiness, feeling of taboo or forbidden acts."
4) "She's the one who's obsessed."
5) "Remain a virgin." (In some people's eyes.)
6) "Avoid pregnancy."

Why do guys love having a finger up their butt?

Some guys really enjoy it because a finger can be the perfect tool for massaging and putting pressure on their prostate while stimulating his muscles as well.

Why are some guys so afraid of receiving anal sex?

The same reason anyone might be afraid of receiving anal sex. They are afraid it will hurt. Or they may worry that it will be messy. Perhaps dealing with sex in an area where there might be poop is not sexy to them. They may have irritable bowel syndrome or chronic constipation and feel like their butt will not be a source of pleasure. And then guys have the sad but misguided fear that if they have anal sex and enjoy it, they might be gay.

If a guy likes to have a finger in his butt should I be worried that he is gay?

Never. He has lots of nerves, strong muscles, and a prostate that may be wildly responsive. That is true for every guy, gay or straight. Don't let society's homophobia stop him from having pleasure in any part of his body or stop you from exploring his body.

How can I convince my guy to let me play with his anus without freaking him out?

I call this syndrome being "butt shy"! There are so many men who are skittish around anything having to do with his butt. There are three possible responses he will give you:

If you slowly warm him up to the idea, he may enjoy anal play with you rather quickly. Or he may say no today but warm up to the idea with time. It could be next week or take two years. But at least you have established the fact that you are open and willing. Or he may never want to go there. Whatever the choice, it's his to make. You have to respect it.

How to Introduce Him to Receiving Anal Sex

Watch his response to your touch around his inner thighs, balls, perineum, and anus. You may see him jump or tense up his muscles. Sometime we think it's fun to tickle our partner and see them jump, but if you want to explore this area of his body you will have to refrain from teasing and tickling him. Your goal is to relax and trust you while you touch these sensitive areas.

If he says he is willing to explore, start with sensual touches. In the normal course of using your hands on his shaft, slide your hand all the way down until you are holding his balls.

With your hand still on his balls, let him know your plans. Say to him, "I want to touch your perineum. I know you are ticklish around there, but I promise I won't tickle you."

If he is agreeable then slide your fingers back to his perineum, using your finger pads to create a rhythmic pressure, or do a firm circular massage on his perineum. Tune in and gauge his response.

Continue to take small steps, maybe go a little further with each encounter the two of you have. Massaging the outside of his anus. Using your tongue on his balls and perineum.

Through the whole process stay tuned in to his response. With a little time and practice he will be able to relax and experience new heights of pleasure with you, around his perineum and elsewhere perhaps! If all goes well, this could be the beginning of him being able to eroticize his butt area and possibly open up his mind to anal play.

How can I convince my partner to have anal sex with her?

You can't. She needs to decide that anal sex is something she is ready for and desiring. You can talk to her about it and let her know you are curious and open to exploring anal sex sometime down the road.

Ask her why she may be hesitating. If she has any fears or concerns, you could share this book or some other great sex guide like *The Ultimate Guide to Anal Sex*, by Tristan Tarimino, with her and see if, as a couple, you can alleviate her fears together.

She may say yes or she may say no. She may think about it for a while and warm up to the idea. Or she may never want to have anal sex. Let her make her choice and then you must respect whatever she decides.

How can I have anal sex without pain?

Let me make one thing very clear: anal sex should never be painful. If it hurts, something is wrong. Your body is giving you a signal. Listen to it. Perhaps you need more lube, a slower stroke, stillness for a few moments, a smaller toy, or maybe you just need to stop and do something else at that moment.

Anal sex, however, can feel odd. It can feel uncomfortable, as if you are pooping backward. But that sensation, once you are acclimated to anal penetration, usually dissipates after a few moments. If it is hurting you, stop. For that matter, anytime *anything* hurts you during sex, stop.

Listen to your body. Breathe. Relax. Assess the situation.

I had anal sex while drunk once, but without being drunk I am terrified of doing it. How can I get over this fear?

If you are determined to try anal play, go slow. Have plenty of lube on hand. Try something small first, like your own finger. Or buy a small butt toy and try penetrating yourself the next time you are masturbating. This will help you get used to the sensation of being penetrated.

When you have anal sex with a partner, be sure your partner is a person you can trust. You need to know that if you tell them to stop, for any reason, they will stop.

I have had anal sex only once and it was very painful and I totally freaked. We were having vaginal sex and supposedly he slipped and penetrated my butt. Will it hurt like that every time?

I am sorry you had a painful experience. That was not anal sex, that was an accident. Satisfying anal sex is done with the intention of finding pleasure for both partners. It is done with verbal consent. You and you partner need to talk about it before beforehand, and let each other know if you are ready to take the plunge.

When done well and experienced under comfortable circumstance anal sex will be pain-free and may feel great for you. Sometimes if you have had a painful experience with anal sex, your body may remember that pain and be unable to relax even if your mind says you are ready to try it again. Again, go slow, breathe, relax, and tune in to your body's signals.

Is it unclean or dangerous to go from vaginal sex to anal sex?

Keep butt play and vaginal play separate. If you take your mouth, finger, toy, penis, or anything and go from butt play to vaginal play you stand a good chance of giving her a vaginal and/or urinary tract an infection. Keep all butt stuff out of her pussy.

In rare cases guys can develop a urinary tract infection from having unprotected anal sex with their partner. Butt bacteria can get into his urethra, too. Ouch.

What diseases can you get from anal sex?

I am a huge advocate for condoms, especially when it comes to anal sex. The thin membranes of the anal area leave us very vulnerable to sexually transmitted diseases (STDs). The STDs that can be contracted through unprotected anal sex include: chlamydia, crabs, gonorrhea, hepatitis B, herpes, HIV, syphilis, warts (HPV), and assorted viruses and parasites that can affect your whole intestinal tract. Honestly, almost every STD known can be passed between partners during anal sex. In fact you don't even have to have penetration to acquire some of these STDs because your condom may not cover the STDs that reside on external skin. These infections can be passed from giver to receiver or the other way around by rubbing skin or on your fingers and hands. To make it even more complex, STDs inside your anal canal can be hard to detect. If that doesn't make you want to protect yourself in every possible way, you need to think again!

What safety precautions could be taken when practicing anal sex?

Make safer sex barriers a priority. Put on a condom. Slip on some gloves. Use a dental dam. Please also remember that sex toys can carry sexually transmitted disease and should be covered with a condom as well.

It's about respecting your own body and respecting your partner's body. A large percentage of people have no idea they are carrying a disease. Not all STDs have symptoms and some can lay dormant in a person's body for years.

You can also take a good look at your partner's body for evidence of any open sores. Sores may be in their body, around the anal or vaginal opening, or on their skin and covered by pubic hair. If you see something that you suspect to be an STD, let your partner know.

Share your concern. Offer to go to the doctor with them to check it out. Care for their body.

How can you assure cleanliness (no poop) during anal sex?

The truth is you can't guarantee absolute cleanliness during anal sex. If you and your partner want to have butt play, you need to remember that poop passes through the anus and that is a simply fact of life.

I have been known to give the following disclaimer before anal sex, "We can have anal sex. I'm into it. But you know what a person uses their butt for. If there's any poop—it's on you!" And then I will roll around laughing. Saying that has always made me feel better. Like I gave them a warning. I gave them a chance to not have to go there. Once they do, they are in for whatever may happen,

If you are having healthy bowel movements and have had one that day, there should be no real mess. There may be what I call "a little residual poop" involved. A smudge, but nothing major.

Some people like to give themselves a warm water enema before anal sex, so they can feel especially clean. Most people however don't have the foresight or desire to do that. If you are having healthy poops, an enema shouldn't be necessary.

Just for peace of mind I recommend buying butt toys that are black in color so if there is a little residue it will not be so obvious. You can also get condoms and latex gloves in black.

If you are not feeling well on a particular day (digestion problems, diarrhea, or constipation) you should avoid anal play and let your body heal. If you are a person who has chronic problems with your digestion or bowel movements you will want to avoid anal play altogether to avoid aggravating your symptoms.

I have heard a person will have trouble pooping after anal sex. Is this true?

Sometimes a person may have trouble pooping after anal sex. Anal sex can be an extreme experience, especially if you are new to it or don't do it very often. Some people say they feel like they have less control over their anal muscles, they report feeling sore or say they cannot hold their bowel movements as long as they could on a day that doesn't involve anal play. With a little time these feelings go away. Some people find it's more than they can deal with and opt not to have anal sex in the future, while others feel like the pleasure they get from anal sex makes a little discomfort worth it.

Does your butt get stretched out from having anal sex?

Nope. If you are having healthy anal sex you do not need to worry about your anus stretching out or that you'll have to wear a diaper or anything like that. Having healthy anal sex can actually be good for your sphincter muscles. It relaxes them, brings circulation through your muscles, and to quote one of my favorite sex educators, Rachel Venning, "it's like doing yoga for your ass!"

The only time I have heard of people injuring these muscles is if they do not or cannot listen to the signals their body is giving them. By signals I mean *pain*. If you feel pain, something is wrong. Stop what you are doing.

There are times when pain signals are blocked, like when you are drunk or high. If you think about it, a drunken person can fall down, skin their knee, and wake up the next morning with no recollection of even having been hurt. Their ability to feel pain is blocked by intoxication. To have healthy anal sex you should be sober and listen to your body, especially if you are new to anal sex.

What is the best position for anal sex?

Most people report they love to do it from behind (doggy-style). The second most favored anal position is with the receiver on their back, legs spread, and knees up (missionary-style.) The best position for you is up to you and your partner to decide. You could try it with the receiving partner leaning over a soft piece of furniture. Or with the giver sitting in a chair and the receiver lowering themself down on top of the giver. Or with the giver lying down on the floor and the receiver squatting over them. Use your imagination and who knows what you may find?

20.

Sex Toys

Sex toys are beautiful. For many of us they bring immense amounts of pleasure, laughter, titillation, joy, and relaxation into our lives. Some people, however, believe sex outside of procreation (makin' babies) is unnatural and sex toys therefore are unnatural, too.

This baffles me. As long as there have been people on earth we have been finding weird things to screw. It's true! Go back in history and you will find myths of women in Polynesia getting knocked up by the bananas they humped. The Chinese grew a tubular plant that they boiled until it was hard enough for them to do 'em. And the ancient Greeks made dildos out of wood and leather. Dildos were so popular in the ancient world there were actual phallic factories and the dildos were exported all over the Mediterranean.

Sex toys are natural and a great way to get off, not to mention have safer sex. Sex toys are remarkable tools for exploring your body and expanding your orgasmic potential. So, read on and learn how you can add more pleasure to your life!

What is a vibrator?

A vibrator is any toy that vibrates. They come in a multitude of shapes, sizes, colors, and textures. Vibrators are most effective on a woman's clit, but once the vibe is yours, you can use it anywhere you like!

Most vibrators run on batteries. Generally, toys that require larger batteries or more than one battery, will have stronger vibrations. A vibrator that plugs into your wall socket will give a more consistent, deep tissue massage. These toys are especially good if you are a woman who has never orgasmed before or has difficulties reaching orgasm.

Is it true that once you use a vibrator, sex just doesn't do it for you? Will a vibrator ruin me for my boyfriend?

No. There is nothing that can replace the wonderful things a lover can do for you. A sex toy is fun but it will never have a heartbeat, write you a love letter, laugh, breathe hot breath into your ear, share breakfast with you, or do your laundry. In other words, you can have a stellar orgasm with your vibrator, but it will never compare to the experiences (sexual or otherwise) you can have with an attentive lover. If your lover cannot give you the kind of orgasm you really desire, then you need to share this book with them; teach them how to expand their skills and possibly how to use your vibrator on you!

If you are a virgin, will using a sex toy ruin sex for you?

Nope. Sex toys can wake up your nerve endings and ultimately make you more orgasmic with and without a partner. Exploring your body is an important step to understanding where and how you find your pleasure. Sex toys can actually help you do that on your own. This way when you have your first sexual encounter with a partner, you will know where to find your pleasure and you will be able to show your partner how to touch you. Keep in mind that your first encounter with a partner may not be as easy as playing with a toy. You will have to be aware of your partner's experience and will need to communicate your needs to her or him. When you do have partnered sex for the first time you may feel nervous, vulnerable, and/or titillation in ways you have never before. Partnered sex can be complex but ultimately well worth it!

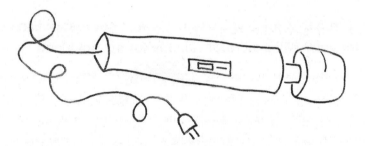

Are there any toys that can guarantee orgasm?

No. There is nothing that can guarantee an orgasm every time you have sex. Sometimes we just don't orgasm. That's normal. If you are a person who has never orgasmed or has trouble orgasming, you may want to try a Hitachi Magic Wand or a Wahl 7-in-1. The strong, deep tissue massaging action of these two toys can wake up nerve endings and inspire orgasms like no other.

> # FACT:
>
> Vibrators that plug in to the wall will almost always have a stronger, deep tissue vibration. Vibrators that have batteries tend to be subtler. It's always best to buy your toy from a boutique-style shop where they have a sample of each product on display with batteries. Then you can hold it in your hand and compare the various toys.

True Tales of Sex Toy Love:

"Having worked at a sex toy shop for years, I'm beyond spoiled in the toy department! I have over thirty vibrators, plus plenty of butt plugs, dildos, bondage and sensation accessories, etc. Truth be told, though, if I had to throw it all away except for one lucky item, I'd be 100 percent fine with just my tried-and-true, trusty ol' Hitachi Magic Wand. I didn't used to be so attached to it; I thought much of the hype surrounding it was, well, nothing but hype. But then my lazy, indecisive self started keeping it plugged in by my bed so it would only take me the second to reach for it to be geared up for a quick fix. This sucker is *strong*. And bulky, yes, but it's easy to lay it down and just get on top of it so you don't have to hold it up. I now use my Magic Wand just about every single day, and about 90 percent of the time it's during sex with my boyfriend. Doggy-style, so it doesn't get in the way. It's magic. Just like its damn name."

" Sex toys are one of my favorite things in life. I own about twenty-five and will never stop collecting. I often get more turned on at the thought of a sex toy than an actual person. I have been known to look at sex toy sites and masturbate thinking about what the toys could do for me. **"**

Which type of textured sex toy provides the most pleasure?

This is something you need to explore for yourself. Each person is unique in how they respond to sex toy design elements like materials, texture, vibration, and size. I recommend buying a couple of different, less expensive toys and exploring how your body responds to each one. For example you might buy a soft rubber vibrating toy and a hard plastic vibrating toy. You might experiment with an egg-shaped vibrator and a phallic-shaped vibrator. You could try a toy with a smooth surface and another with bumps. If you are using your toy for penetration, a smooth toy will give you a faster stroke while a curvy toy gives your muscles something to work around. Use each toy inside your body, outside your body, with vibration, without vibration, use the toys together, use the toys alone, with a partner, without a partner—really test every possibility! I suggest buying less expensive toys because if you do not know exactly what you like, it's easier to define your preferences when you buy a bunch of very different toys. Once you know what you like, then seek out high-quality products that match your preferences. Exploring sex toys and your body is an ongoing, super fun way to grow sexually.

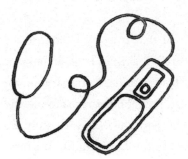

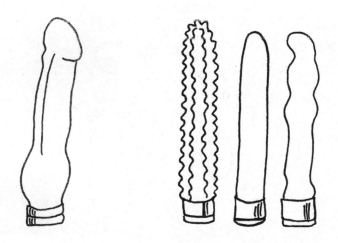

My Latest Discovery

One of the many great things about working at Babeland was the employee discount. I bought everything I ever wanted to try! I screwed my way through every vibrator, dildo, butt toy, blindfold, cock ring, condom, lube, cream, game, and any other item that tickled my interest! And the best part? I never got tired of trying something new and never stopped finding new and exciting items. I still don't.

A perfect example of that is a toy I found the other day called Reckless Rabbit. This rabbit is what I call an "add-on." You can slide it onto another toy or have your partner wear it on their cock. During vaginal penetrative play, the rabbit curves around the receiver's pubic bone while the little bump on the other side stimulates her perineum and butt. What looked to me like a funny curiosity ended up being very orgasmic!

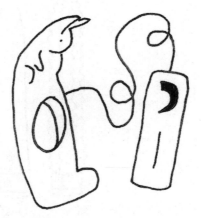

What is the best toy to travel with?

You can travel with any toy. If you are flying just be sure to take the batteries out before you pack it. It's a real drag to have your bag pulled off an airplane and destroyed by a bomb-defusing robot just because you forgot to take the batteries out of your vibrator!

If you worry about baggage security seeing your toy, you shouldn't. When I travel to do presentations, I frequently bring toy samples with me and sometimes I pack dozens of sex toys! This will often flag a baggage security officer's curiosity. They have never pulled a toy out of my bag for inspection. When asked about the items I just say, "That's a toy." They usually respond with, "Oh. OK." Most security officers are polite about these things.

Here's another tip: pack toys in the luggage you are checking rather than in your carry-on luggage. This way if they do check your luggage it is most often not in your presence so you do not even have to answer to them.

Once at your destination you may have other travel toy concerns. Look for more silent toys, as they can provide more discretion if you are staying somewhere where you do not want people to know your business, like at a family member's home. If you are sharing a hotel room with someone and want privacy, toss a waterproof toy into your toiletry bag and have your fun in the shower!

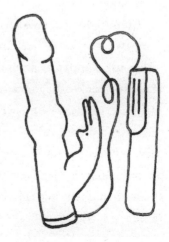

What is The Rabbit?

There are many toys on the market today with the rabbit name. The toy comes in various rabbit shapes, but a company called Vibrotex invented the original Rabbit Habit. The Rabbit Habit is a dual action vibrator. It has a shaft that goes inside a woman's vagina and an extra vibrating branch that curves over her vulva and stimulates her clit at the same time. It is called "The Rabbit Habit" because the clit-tickler is shaped like a little bunny with two firm ears that flicker around the clit when the vibrator is turn on.

Vibrotex is a Japanese company that has since become famous for their very thoughtful, high-quality, and unique sex toy creations. They built this toy in the rabbit shape because in Japan it is illegal to manufacture any product in the shape of a penis. They managed to skirt this law by making what would be the shaft of the penis look like a little man with a helmet of hair to emulate the head of the penis and the external vibrating piece in the shape of a bunny.

Admittedly it is an odd-looking toy, but so effective that no one cares what it looks like! In fact, the toy became so popular that other toy companies around the world started creating all sorts of Rabbit knock-offs and adding animal shapes like monkeys and dolphins to many of their other products. And you thought it was just that women had a kinky attraction to rabbits? Nope. We just have a kinky attraction to quality! Speaking of which, I will always recommend the Japanese toys over any other products because their manufacturing standards tend to be higher than those of other countries.

Why are some sex toys so unattractive?

Beauty is always a matter of opinion, but even I, a lover of sex toys, will admit there are some really ugly sex toys out there. Luckily, there are such a wide variety of products available today that if you search, you can find something that will match your taste.

The toys I find to be especially unattractive are the realistic dildos in fleshy colors. Sometimes the manufacturers will go to great lengths to make color variations between the head and shaft and even paint veins down the underside. Whenever I see one of these toys, I feel like I am looking at a severed body part.

I prefer my toys to be in bright candy colors or leopard print to match my bedsheets. I love beautiful curved glass butt plugs, stainless steel vibrators, kooky-looking dongs from outer space, soft fuzzy cuffs, and peacock feather ticklers. I could go on and on.

Ultimately I just want my toys to look like toys, not body parts. But my experience working in a sex toy boutique has taught me that other individuals love love love those veiny, fleshy realistic dongs, with all their heart—as much as I love my candy-colored g-spotters. They want something that looks and feels as close to the real thing as possible. Who am I to deny them that pleasure? I learned that just because a toy does not spark my passion that does not mean it won't appeal to anyone else. If you see a sex toy that turns you off, keep looking and you may find just the thing for you!

Why are some sex toys so expensive?

For the most part the more expensive toys are imported from Japan or made by small companies that have high overheads and high manufacturing standards. The less expensive toys are made in China by companies that look to sell quantity over quality. In many cases you get what you pay for.

If you have a limited income there are many great options for you. The Silver Bullet is generally the least expensive toy. But it's a great vibrator. Plus, there are always items around your house that can bring you oodles of pleasure. Your tub faucet can be loads of fun. Just find a mild temperature and scoot your butt right under the running water, letting the flow of water hit your vulva. This is totally fun! Use your silk stockings as a sweet blindfold. Go to the hardware shop and find soft rope and eyehooks for a little bondage play. Clothespins make great nipple clips. Ice cubes create some amazing sensation play. Use your imagination and the possibilities are all around you and totally affordable.

Can a vibrator be too strong?

Absolutely. If a vibrator feels too strong, it can overstimulate your nerve endings and feel irritating. The only true way to know how your body will react to a particular toy is to try it. However, due to the nature of these products, taking a sex toy on a test drive is simply not possible. For this reason I recommend buying your vibrator from a sex toy boutique where they have sample models out on display. Then you can turn it on, hold it in your hand, and get a pretty good idea how strong or subtle the vibration is. If you do not have a sex toy boutique of this nature in your city then you should hire one of the many sex toy home party companies to do a party for you and your friends. It's a great way to see the items up close and understand exactly what you are buying.

I also recommend looking for sex toys that have variable speeds rather than just one speed. Vibrators with variable speeds will have a dial switch or set of buttons that you turn to make the vibration go from low to high. Then you can adjust the speed to fit your body's needs at that moment.

— · — · —

Sex Toy Home Parties

One of the most fun ways to be introduced to the various products on the market is to book a sex toy home party. It's a great way to pull your friends together, have some laughs, and learn. Check the Resources at the back of this book for a listing of sex toy home party companies that have great reputations and fantastic products. They have representatives in big cities, small towns down South, and even internationally! In most cases, if you have a party at your home there are all sorts of incentives like *free sex toys!*

Can your clitoris get sore from using a vibrator too much?

Yes. Some women need an extreme amount of pressure on their clit in order to orgasm. She can apply so much pressure with a vibrator or other hard surface that she may cause bruising, inflammation, or even tear the delicate vulva tissue. If this happens to you, you should leave your clit alone until the soreness subsides and use less pressure in the future. If you tear tissue you will need to assess the damage and possibly see a doctor. I always recommend using lube with your vibrator, even if you are only using your vibe on your vulva and not inside your body, just to protect your tissue and cut down on friction.

I need a tremendous amount of pressure on my clitoral area to achieve orgasm, such as a hard piece of wood like a table edge. Are there any sex toys that might be able to work my clit like this?

The Hitachi Magic Wand. On high speed it has been compared to a freaking jackhammer! (By me anyway.) However, it still has a softer, round head that will be easy on your body. If you get one and find it is too strong for your body, use the lower speed and use it through your jeans, blanket, or with a washcloth over your clit, just to soften the sensation.

How do I approach my spouse about sex toys without making him feel insecure?

Tell your spouse the truth. If you have never used a sex toy, let him or her know you are curious about them. Explain that you want to share your pleasure with him/her. If you see a toy that interests you online, print out a photo of it and show it to your partner. You might say, "Hey, doesn't this look cool?" or "I am so curious! We should buy one and see what it does." Be confident with your idea and make it a fun event that the two of you can share. Wanting to share your sex toy play with your partner is normal and healthy.

You may also want to share this book with your spouse. Pull it out one night after a fun bout of sex and explore it together. Point out the things he already does that drive you wild. Build his confidence. Then find a picture of a sex toy you think might be fun and point it out.

For a holiday, you might want to buy your lover a gift certificate from a sex toy boutique and then plan a date to go shopping together. When you speak in positives and make sex toys an adventure for the two of you to explore, your spouse might surprise you!

True Tales of Sharing Sex Toys (Or Not):

"I like to use toys with my lovers. It doesn't always come up unless the toys are in arm's reach. Most times, you just have to put it out there, and say hey, let's give this a try. It's all about being assertive as well as respectful."

"Men love power tools and I've yet to find an exception when it comes to sex power tools! Sometimes, with some less experienced guys, it takes a little talking to them to let them know that toys are not a substitute or a replacement for them. This was the case with my fiancé, and while we are both young, he's a little younger and less experienced than I. I let him know that these were here to enhance the experience for the both of us, and basically it gives him even more to play with! He's had tons of fun trying them out on me, and has even been playing with them himself."

"I prefer to keep my toys private. I like the idea of having control over my pleasure whenever I want to. They're mine and I don't share."

> **❝** I am pretty direct. I just tell my partner, 'This is my little bullet. I like to use it during sex because it helps me orgasm. So I will be using it when we have sex, OK?' There's no reason for him to feel inadequate. It's just what I need. **❞**

"I use my toys with my lover and have used toys with several other lovers in the past. I usually talk about my toys before I introduce them, although sometimes I will bring out my cordless bullet during sex first just because it's so nonthreatening. I've never found anyone who didn't enjoy that addition. Usually they like to see me using the toys as much as I like to use them. They get excited about the toys and start asking me to bring them out."

Can I use my vibrator on my guy?

Absolutely! Ask him if he's into it. If he is shy, start by using your vibrator as a back massager to relax him, letting him get used to the sensation, and then move the vibration on to more erogenous zones. Run the toy over his nipples, inner thighs, shaft, head, perineum, and outer butt, and then, if he is into it, put a vibe in his butt. (If you do use a vibe for anal play, be sure you use lube and that your toy has a flared base to prevent it from slipping in past his sphincter muscles and up his butt. Review Chapter 19 for safe and fun anal sex instructions.) Start with a low vibration, and if he likes it work up to something stronger.

If you are sharing your toy with your partner be sure you cover it with a condom. Bacteria and STDs can be passed between partners when sharing toys.

I want to surprise my girlfriend with a sex toy. How do I pick one out for her?

I recommend you buy her a gift certificate from your favorite store or Web site. Most women like to pick their own toys. They know their bodies in ways that are hard to articulate. If there is a nice sex toy shop in your area, then the two of you can go shopping together and make a whole night of it. Super fun! If there is not a nice shop near you, then check out the Resources at the back of this book and buy a gift certificate from an online shop. Then the two of you can log on and explore together!

Do g-spot toys really work and, if so, how do I use one?

Yes. Many women have their first g-spot orgasm with the help of a sex toy specifically designed for g-spotting. G-spotters are usually phallic in shape but have a dramatically curved tip. The g-spot responds to a strong massaging action and the firmer the tip of the g-spotter, the more stimulation you will get out of it.

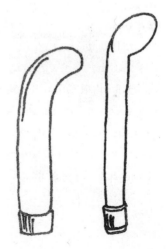

Often the g-spotting toys will be as long as eight inches. If you insert the full length of the toy, you will be stimulating her cervix and that it not the spot. Her g-spot is located at the opening of her pussy, no deeper than two inches. Insert the g-spotter into the opening of her vagina, with the curve pointed toward her naval, about one and a half to two inches inside. No matter how long the toy may be, think of the part of the toy that is outside her body as the handle. Most often we use an insertable toy with an in-out motion, but this is not how you get great g-spot stimulation. Instead, use the handle to rock the toy up and down to create a massaging motion.

Some women like vibration on their g-spot and others do not. If you do not know what you like, I recommend buying a vibrating g-spotter because you can always just turn it off.

Why can I only have a g-spot orgasm with my Nubby G?

The g-spot can be a finicky thing. For some women it can be very hit-or-miss. They may never feel anything in that area, while other women find it downright annoying to have their g-spot stimulated. If you have found a toy, a movement, or position that works, go for it! It could be that for you the Nubby G has just the right girth, tip shape, firmness, or level of vibration. Explore other g-spotters with similar features and see if you can find the element that is sparking for you. If for some reason you cannot figure it out, you always have your Nubby G!

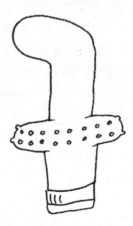

True Tales of G-spotting:

"A lot of women have mainly clitoral orgasms, but I tend to have more internal g-spot orgasms, and a tiny little vibe isn't going to do it for me. This is usually due to the fact that it's difficult to find many "soft" toys that can deliver decent vibration, as well as good reach, pressure, and leverage necessary for me to access my g-spot properly."

"My absolute favorite sex toy is the Archer Wand. It seriously feels like it was made for my body specifically. It's very simple in design, but does exactly what I need. One ball hits my g-spot while the other hits my clit. It's glass so it warms up to my body right away, which feels very nice. It's smooth. I was never one that liked textured things in my vagina. And above all it makes me ejaculate a lot. I soak through several towels. Lovers of mine that really like to see me get wet love to play with this toy."

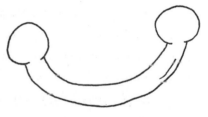

Sex Toy Buyer Beware

There are no agencies in existence that govern the manufacturing, package labeling, or advertising standards of any sex toys, lubes, and lotions. Consequently some sex toys are better than others. They may have better or worse manufacturing qualities. They may or may not have a manufacturer's warranty. They may be made with materials that you are allergic to. They may have deceptive package labeling. It's up to you to be a discerning customer. You need to take responsibility for finding toys that are good for your body. What can you do to protect yourself?

- Shop from an online boutique or storefront boutique where the people will honestly answer your questions and accept returns on defective or substandard products.

- After you purchase your product open it up in the shop. Check toys with plastic casings to ensure they have smooth edges and sealed seams. If your toy is jelly/rubber look for obvious bubbles or flaws in the rubber that may make your toy vulnerable to rips and tears.

- Ask the store clerk to lend you a set of batteries so you can be sure the motor works.
- If you get the product home and you find the lube or lotion you purchased makes your skin burn or become

inflamed, discontinue using it. You may be having an allergic reaction.

- If you are allergic to latex, be aware that there is latex in many soft jelly/rubber toys.

- If your toy has a distinct "new" smell it is probably made with industrial chemicals that may cause skin inflammation for some. Wash the toy, let it air out, and cover it with a condom when you use it. Throw it out if it bothers your skin. Try toys that have been constructed with an alternative material like hard plastic, metal, glass, or latex.

- I always recommend tasting your new sex toy. (I'm an animal!) The membranes in your mouth are very similar to the membranes in a woman's vulva and vagina. If it tastes bad or makes your tongue tingle, I would follow the directions above or possibly pass on it altogether.

What is a dildo?

A dildo is anything that is phallic-shaped. A dildo can be made out of solid materials like plastic, rubber, wood, metal, or stone. A cucumber or a banana can work as a dildo, although I don't recommend using them unless you're sure they have no sharp edges and you have washed them and slipped them inside a condom. A vibrator that is shaped like a cock is a vibrating dildo. As I said, anything that is more or less shaped like a cock can be a dildo.

There are oodles of variations of dildos out there. I think the best

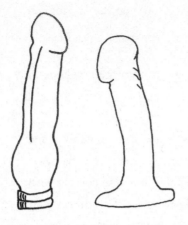

dildos on the market today are made of silicone. Silicone dildos (unlike jelly/rubber or plastic dildos) are nonporous. This means they do not have the microscopic pores that the other materials tend to have. They do not harbor bacteria and can be thoroughly cleaned in a pot of boiling water or on the top rack of your dishwasher. (There really is something so sweet about walking into a friend's house and finding their sex toys drying in the dish rack or bubbling in a pot of hot water!)

One type of dildo people really love is the suction-cup dildo. These novel toys have a suction-cup base so you can attach it to any hard surface, like your refrigerator door, the tile in your shower or the seat of a folding chair. Making it possible for you to find fun ways to have sex in totally new places and positions!

Is bigger always better when it comes to a dildo?

Not always. Size is relative to the individual. Some people crave a large dildo while others may, for any number of reasons, need a smaller one. It's all about how *you* respond to size.

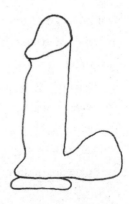

How do you choose a dildo?

I always recommend comparing them to the size of your hand. Your hands are used during sex play all the time. Consequently, hands are a great guide to size and extremely convenient because they are always with you! If you know your body can accommodate three fingers, then find a toy that matches the width of your three fingers.

While in the sex toy shop take a few moments and think about what toys or tools your body has really responded positively to in the past and try to match them. Look at the length of the dildo with the same kind of contemplation.

Other things to consider are whether you want a realistic-shaped toy or not. Do you want a toy with an extreme curve to massage your g-spot or prostate? Do you want a smooth surface for fast and slick strokes? Or do you want a more bumpy texture so you can feel the grooves as you work your muscles? Really think about your body and what you have enjoyed in the past and what you want to try.

Be adventurous. If something looks intriguing you might give it a try. You only live once and I believe you ought to be able to have every fun experience you possibly can!

Are glass dildos safe?

A beautiful glass toy is smooth and sensual. It warms up with your body or can be popped in the refrigerator for some cool sensation play. The material is so solid that it will not crack in your hands. But it is glass and consequently can shatter if dropped. I recommend that before you use a glass toy on yourself or a partner you inspect it. Look for any nicks in the glass, hold it up to light and look for cracks, run your hands across the surface to ensure it is smooth and intact.

Glass toys are as safe as any sex toy. As with silicone or plastic toys, be conscious of what condition your glass dildo is in. Questions you might ask when examining your sex toys include: Is it clean? Are there any defects or cracks? If the toy vibrates, is it overheating? If it plugs in, is the electrical cord intact? Inspecting all of your sex toys is an important part of taking care of your body.

Why do people need lube?

A great lube makes it possible to have longer, more exuberant bouts of sex. But beyond the slippery fun it creates, it's also a great addition to your safer sex plan. Lube cuts down on friction that can cause microscopic abrasions. These abrasions leave you more vulnerable to sexually transmitted diseases and bacterial infections. Lube helps you have safer sex.

When you are shopping for lube, read the ingredients list and get familiar with what you are using. I usually look for the water-based lube with the simplest ingredients list and fewest chemicals because I want to understand what I am using in my body. For my body I avoid glycerin and alcohol. Both of these ingredients irritate my body.

Water-based lubes are safe to use with latex. You will find they vary in consistency; some are thick and gooey while others are thin and watery. Lube manufacturers create lubes with various consistencies to meet the preferences of different people. Pick up a bottle, turn it upside down, and see how runny it is. Pick the product that you think will be the most fun. My favorite water-based lube is *Slippery Stuff*.

The alternative to a water-based lube is silicone lube. Silicone-based lubes are more expensive but well worth the price. A little bit goes a long way. Beyond penetrative play, silicone lubes are great for any skin-on-skin contact—like massages and hand jobs. Silicone lubes are also safe to use with latex, but because they aren't water-based you can use them in the shower or hot tub! (A woman's natural lubrication tends to rinse away if she is playing in water.) When it comes to silicone lubes, I love *i Lube* and *Eros.*

Avoid using things like baby oil or Vaseline for sex play. Oils and petroleum-based products can damage your latex barrier (break your condom). Plus, baby oil has fragrance that can be irritating, especially if used inside a woman's body.

Please remember that lube is a *must* during anal sex. The butt is not self-lubricating like a vagina.

HOMEWORK:

Put a little lube inside his condom so he can feel wetness with the warmth of your body. Also, use a little lube on your fingers and hands when you put them on or in your lover. For the ultimate in slippery, smooth, safe hand-sex wear a well-fitted latex glove drizzled with lube.

Is lubrication bad for you?

No. When you find the right lube for your body it is actually good for you. But lube is like any personal product so exploring your options is essential. For example, your best friend may find a lube that they love but when you try it you may find their favorite lube is too sticky, too watery, or even itchy and irritating for you. When possible buy various small bottles or sampler pillows of lube and compare products. Find the right product for you. If you have a new lover, it may mean changing and finding the product that works for the two of you.

MYTH:

It's a common myth that if a woman is wet she is turned on. But many women can be totally hot to trot and still be dry. Drinking water is a great way to boost your body's natural wetness, but lube is the ultimate way to make sure your fun is always slippery!

Is there any way to keep my lube from drying out and getting sticky?

It sounds like you are using a water-based lube with a sizable amount of glycerin in it. Glycerin gives lube a great consistency but ultimately does dry out. You could change to a silicone-based lube, which contains no glycerin. Or you could keep a spray bottle of water near your bed and reinvigorate your lube with a quick spritz of water. I have heard a number of people say this keeps their lube slippery and the water can add an exciting boost in the middle of their sex play!

What types of lube are safe to use with sex toys?

Water-based lubes will be compatible with every toy and are the easiest to clean up. Silicone lubes can be great for sex play and massage but will not be compatible with silicone-based toys. The understanding among toy retailers is that the two different kinds of silicone—lube being liquid, toys being solid—when combined, try to bond with each other. There is no evidence this will harm you in any way, but it can cause funny silicone nubs to form on your toy, ultimately ruining it. Once while working at Babeland we took a few different silicone toys and soaked them in a bag of silicone lube. Only one of the toys developed these lube nubs. But when you are paying upward of fifty dollars for a fine silicone sex toy, you don't want to risk ruining it. When in doubt, slap a condom on your toy and use any lube you like!

How to Clean Your Sex Toys

There are many sex toy cleaning products. They are not necessary but can be convenient, unless you are sensitive to fragrance and chemicals. First determine what your toy is made out of and then follow these simple instructions.

All Toys: If you plan on sharing your sex toy with a partner, always cover it with a condom. I will often put a condom on my toy just so I am sure it's clean and safe for my body. When you wash your toys, be sure they are completely dry before you put them away. According to the Goodvibes.com, most bacteria and viruses cannot survive on a dry surface. I recommend storing your toys in covered plastic bins or plastic zip bags. Zip bags are great if you share a toy box with your lover. You can label your bags and/or designate which toys are for vaginal use only, as you never want to use an anal toy for vaginal play without covering it with a condom first because anal bacteria can cause vaginal infections. If you have numerous toys, you may want to bag them just to keep them from resting on each other. Jelly/rubber toys will sometimes deteriorate faster if they are touching other rubber or plastic toys.

Vibrators: If it is waterproof lather it up with a little mild soap and rinse it thoroughly under the faucet. If it is not waterproof wipe it down with a soapy washcloth and rinse with a wet washcloth. You can also wipe it down with cotton and a small amount of rubbing alcohol just to remove any soap residue. Again, unless your toy is waterproof, you cannot get the battery pack wet. When in doubt, assume your toys are not waterproof.

Silicone: Wash with warm water and soap. Silicone toys are nonporous and therefore harbor less bacteria than a jelly/rubber or plastic toy. If your toy does not have a motor, you can even drop it in a pot of boiling water for ten minutes to really give it a good cleaning from time to time. Silicone toys transfer heat so be sure to let it cool off before you touch your toy.

Jelly/Rubber: If they do not vibrate, then simply lather them up with a mild soap and rinse under water. If they have a motor, then follow the vibrator instructions above.

Cyber skin or Softskin: These superrealistic toys are a big hit for people who are looking for a true flesh feeling. They do however require a bit more care than your average toy. Wash your toy with soap and water as you would a jelly/rubber or vibrating toy. Dry it with a paper towel. Then powder it with cornstarch. (I recommend you do not use talc because for a number of years it has been suspected as a potential risk factor for ovarian cancer.) If you do not powder your cyber skin toy it will get sticky and collect lint and hair.

Leather and Vinyl: You cannot sanitize these materials. To give them a basic cleaning, wash your item with a soapy washcloth and towel dry.

Nylon and Fabric: Hand-wash in the sink and lay flat to dry.

Why would a woman want to wear a strap-on harness?

I never understood why a woman would want to wear a harness—or how amazing they can be—until I strapped one on. I am very femme and full of pussy pride. I had never even fantasized about having a cock or using my hips to be that kind of driving force with my lovers. Plus I have a big butt and full hips. Almost all of my clothes have to be tailored to fit me; how was this one-size-fits-all thing going to look and feel on me?

On one of my first days working at Babeland I was going through product knowledge training with my friend Dana. She insisted that I try on a couple of harnesses over my jeans just so I would understand how they work and how to fit customers. Lo and behold, after a couple of tries, I found the perfect harness—The Bionic Two-Strap in blue-sparkle vinyl!

This harness works for me for many reasons.

- *Fun.* I did not understand how playful a harness could be. The blue-sparkle vinyl made me feel like a superhero!
- *Femme.* I felt like the sparkle also gave my harness a cool femme appeal. It matched perfectly my blue, full-length sequin dress!
- *Fit.* It fit my round butt because the two-strap feature fits like a jock strap. You can fit the biggest or the smallest butt between those adjustable straps with such ease. Finally, it simply felt sexy.
- *Function.* The hole in the center enabled me to pop any toy with a flared base into my harness and have my way with the world. Of course I picked out a blue-sparkle silicone dildo—I'm into matching!

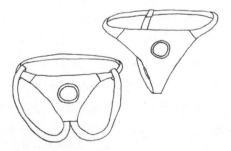

How do I pick the right harness for my body?

I like the two-strap harness but you may prefer a one-strap, which fits like a thong. Some women like the feel of leather over their vulva. I prefer the two-strap however because it allows me to touch and reach most of my vulva if I want to. Some people find they have more control over their dildo wearing a one-strap, while others find the two-strap gives them more control.

No matter what kind of harness you wear, your clit will be stimulated with every thrust if you position the base of your dildo to press up against it. With the right dildo base you'll even get a little suction action on your clit!

Beyond straps, you should consider the type of material your harness is made from. You can choose from materials like vinyl, rubber, leather, and velvet. Again, selection is all about personal choice. Some people like soft leather because with time it forms to your body and soon fits like a glove. Other people prefer rubber because you can play in the shower with rubber and easily clean it.

When purchasing a harness, look at the buckles, too. Some people like a standard buckle because it stays in place, other people like a D-ring buckle because you can tighten or loosen your harness with ease while you are wearing it.

Finally, you will want to look at the hole that your dildo fits in. Some are a fixed size and will limit the size of dick you can wear while others are adjustable.

Another harness that I find to be pretty cool and creative is the thigh harness. This simple harness fits most flare-based toys and then straps around your thigh, a pillow, a chair, or maybe even a tree trunk! Get creative with it and the list of possibilities is endless!

Why are harnesses such elaborate contraptions?

Once you have tried on a harness, it will make a lot more sense. They have what looks like a lot of straps and buckles, but they're there so you can adjust your harness to fit your body perfectly. Fit is extremely important. The better your harness fits, the more control you will have with your cock. So go to your local sex toy shop and ask if you can try on a harness over your pants.

If you are a larger person, don't be shy about getting a harness. Many of the harnesses out there will fit you, and some of the companies now make extended straps. Call or visit one of the sex toy boutiques I have listed in the Resources section at the back of this book and the salespeople will happily fit you.

If you are a guy looking for a harness, these shops are also a great resource for you. Lots of guys who have had prostate cancer or other ailments that limit their ability to have an erection will enjoy a harness. While working at the sex toy boutique I loved fitting guys for harnesses because these guys were the sweetest. They just want to harness up and please their lovers. You have to respect that!

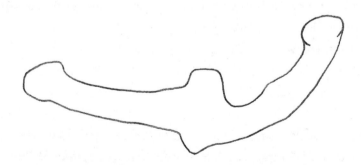

— ∎ — ∎ —

True Tale of Harnesses in Action:

"I believe no woman's sex toy ensemble is complete without a harness! The nicest thing about the harness is that your partner can choose from a multitude of toys to go with it. Depending on the mood, you can accent your harness with a dildo that is long or short, thick or thin, vibrating or nonvibrating. Moreover, getting head while wearing the harness (particularly with a Nexus dildo) can be a special treat!"

Is it normal for guys to like it when girls use strap-ons on them? I love the idea of my girl riding my wagon, if you know what I mean. I want to receive a good fucking by a woman with a strap-on! Am I normal?

It's your ass, so go for it! I believe many people are afraid to admit (even to their lover) their true desires. It takes a real man to pony up and take it in the butt. In fact, it's so common that there are a few great adult videos on the subject. Check out the video *Bend Over Boyfriend* for some inspiration!

HOMEWORK:

It is currently illegal to purchase sex toys in Alabama, Georgia, Kansas, Louisiana, Mississippi, Texas, and Virginia. This issue is larger than you might think. What may look like an absurd case of a few southern states' conservative governments being scared of vibrating rubber doodads is actually a frightening case of the government seeping into our basic rights of privacy. The court's decision to uphold these laws can set a precedent that can be used to create and uphold other laws that will affect everyone's sexual freedoms.

How do they pass these laws? The silence of citizens. Lawmakers are sure that shame and fear will keep us from admitting that we buy and enjoy sex toys. The more you speak shamelessly of sex toys as a positive force, the closer we will get to living in a more honest and sex-positive society. Your mission? Drop any embarrassment you may feel so that the next time someone cracks a joke about a dildo you can simply say, "I have a dildo and I love it." Like it's no big deal. Because it isn't.

You can log on and take a stand on important sexual issues by visiting freespeechcoalition.com.

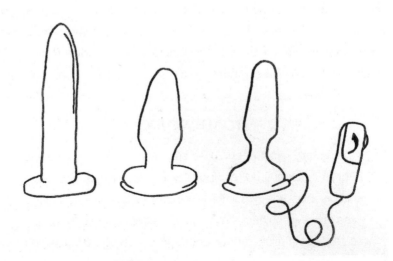

What is a butt plug?

A butt plug is exactly what it sounds like: a toy that is inserted in your butt and has a flared base to keep it from slipping past your sphincter muscles. Some butt plugs have an indentation at the base. These plugs are meant to slip in and stay in place, creating what can be some very pleasurable pressure in the butt muscles. Other butt plugs are smooth from top to base and have no indentation. These toys are meant to move in and out of the butt, a sensation that can also be very exciting.

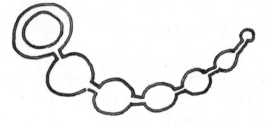

How do you use anal beads?

Anal beads can be fun for the beginner and the experienced butt-sex lover alike because they give your muscles a chance to relax in between inserting each bead. Use lube, pop a bead in, relax, breathe, pop another bead in, and so on. Once the beads are in you can have any kind of sex play you like, including oral sex, clitoral stimulation, or vaginal penetration. When the bead-wearer is about to orgasm, gently begin to pull the beads out. For many people this sensation on their sphincter muscles will inspire a stronger, muscular orgasm.

I recommend buying solid silicone or rubber beads that are

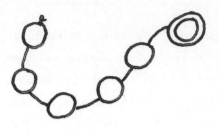

connected together as one piece as apposed to the plastic beads that are tied together with a string. The string beads are inexpensive, but impossible to clean. You will have to throw them out after one use. Also I have heard too many tales of people getting slight friction burns from the string as they pull it out or even scratched by the cheap plastic beads. Ouch! I don't want you to scratch your very sensitive butt.

Can I use my vibrator in my butt?

Vibrators can feel amazing on the outside of the asshole and really help warm you up for penetration. Almost any vibrator can be used on the outside of the butt. If you are going to use a vibe inside your body, again, be sure it has a flared base.

I cannot begin to tell you how important it is that every toy you ever put in your butt or your lover's butt has a flared base of some kind. If the toy or object you use does not have a flared base, it can very easily slip past the strong anal muscles and get stuck inside a person.

The tissue in your butt is very soft and delicate and can easily wrap around a "lost" toy. If you try to simply push the toy out you will feel pain and possibly damage the delicate tissue inside your butt.

I also recommend covering your vibrator with a condom. You never want to introduce any residue from the butt into her pussy because that can cause a mean urinary tract infection.

How far can a person penetrate anally?

A person's rectum is about five inches long but does have very soft walls that sort of turn and fold around. I would not recommend using toys that are longer than about five inches. Be sure that your enter and exit slowly and use lots of lube.

What is a cock ring?

Cock rings come in many forms, like the stretchy rubber rings, solid aluminum rings, adjustable leather straps with snaps, denim with Velcro fasteners, and so on. But essentially they are all rings, some adjustable and some not.

How does a cock ring work?

His entire package goes into the ring—yes, his penis and his balls—
so that the cock ring sits up against his body. The ring creates a tight
grip at the base of his cock and balls.

Usually when I am describing this to a group of people some of
them will lean in with great interest. Others will squeal and wince
with the realization that the *whole* package goes in the ring. They
assume that this can't possibly be comfortable for the guy. As with
everything it depends upon the guy. This is why so many of the cock
rings are adjustable; every guy responds in his own unique way. If you
have never used a cock ring I strongly suggest you start with one
that's very stretchy or adjustable.

For the best effect, he needs to be erect or semierect when you put
the ring on. If you are using a rubber ring, you may want to use a
little lube on the ring so it does not tug at his hair.

When you refer back to the male anatomy lesson I gave in
Chapter 10 you will realize that the cock ring is gripping some of the
erectile tissue that runs from the base of his cock to his perineum.
This alone is a great sensation for most guys. Beyond that, the cock
ring is also restricting the veins that allow blood to flow out of his
penis. So more blood is flowing in than out. This is going to engorge
his blood vessels. He will have these subtle but amazing sensations
that he is harder and bigger. (Sorry, you are not actually bigger
guys—you just feel that way!) Ultimately it will take him longer to
orgasm and his orgasm will be more intense.

Do cock rings really keep guys harder longer?

For most guys, yes. It can be a good tool to help him maintain his
erection if he is having difficulties in that department. You might

MYTH:

There are stories that float around about a guy who uses a cock ring, gets his penis stuck, and has to go to the emergency room to have the cock ring removed. This scenario does not happen to most cock ring users, but certainly can happen if you use a solid cock ring and do not follow my simple instructions.

Do not use the solid metal cock rings. Use only the easy-to-release stretchy, snap, or Velcro styles.

If a guy has no experience and uses a solid metal cock right he may find it feels too tight and he cannot just take it off immediately. (Like he could if he were using an easy-to-release cock ring.) And then things start to unravel. He panics. His heart beats faster, forcing more blood into his cock. Making it more impossible to get out of the cock ring and making him panic even more. Some guys will get so scared that they will go to the emergency room and have the difficult experience of having the cock ring removed by a doctor.

If you do use a solid cock ring and start to panic, what you want to do is relax. Take deep breaths. Take a cool bath. Do anything you can to slow your heartbeat and bring your erection down.

If you do feel like you need to see a doctor, then just go. Emergency room doctors see sex trauma patients all the time. Maybe not as often as they see people who have had other accidents, but chances are you will not be their first and you will not be their last. Swallow your pride and take comfort in the fact that by law they must keep your privacy.

When using a cock ring, please remember that you are playing with blood flow in the body and always need to be aware of the length of time you or your partner have been wearing the cock ring. I recommend wearing it for no more than twenty minutes. If you wear it for an extended length of time the blood vessels may become too engorged and you'll stand a risk of bursting blood vessels. This is rare, but real. The only case of an injury of this nature I have ever heard of was when a guy was using his cock ring while very drunk and then passed out for many hours while wearing it. Ouch. Follow my advice and you should find nothing but pleasure with your cock ring.

also want try to reduce the amount of stress in your lives. Everyone experiences stress, but when stress persists, the body begins to break down and problems, like erectile dysfunction, can occur.

Are cock rings pleasurable for both partners?

To be honest I did not think a cock ring would do anything for me. I figured I would use it to manipulate my guy's orgasmic experience and find added boost by watching him enjoy something different. But once he had it on and we were having sex I was surprised to find that because the cock ring went around his cock and balls it was pushing more of his body forward and I could feel more of him against my vulva. It was a subtle but pleasant thing!

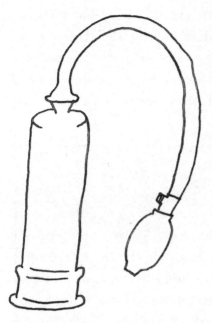

What is a pump?

A pump is a Lucite tube with a pumping device on the end. Sometimes a pump will have a soft inner sleeve, sometimes not. There are penis pumps, clit pumps, and nipple pumps. Use a little lube on the edge of the Lucite container just to create a seal, put your body part of choice inside, and pump the end. This causes hyperemia; simply put, an increase in the quantity of blood flow to that body part. Your blood vessels become engorged and this can be very stimulating. It's a lot like giving your penis, clit, or nipples a hickey! As with any toy that plays with suction and/or blood flow, follow the directions carefully.

While you are in the pump department, be sure to check out some of the toys that are built just for guys. Masturbation sleeves can be a blast. A sleeve is a simple soft jelly/rubber tube or sometimes they are molded to look like a mouth, pussy, or butt. You can submerge a sleeve in hot water to warm it up, add lube, and have the wet, warm sensation that really takes a guy over the edge!

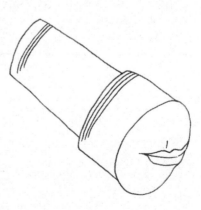

I have never heard more rave reviews for a boy toy than I have for the Flesh Light. It looks like an industrial flashlight. Screw off the cap and there is a super soft, cyberskin sleeve where he inserts his cock. I recommend he use lube for extra sensation. You can unscrew the bottom and drop a vibrator in the end for even more sensation. Plus the sleeve pops right out and can be cleaned in the sink.

MYTH:

For decades companies have been selling penis pumps as "penis enlargement" devices. Unfortunately for many customers, this is all made up. There is no federal administration set up to ensure that sex toy companies are telling the truth in advertisement or on their packages. Therefore any company looking to sell an extra million of their product will slap "penis enlarger" on the package and collect your money. So despite what the package says, a penis pump will never, ever enlarge your penis. At best your cock will look a bit larger while in the device, but as soon as you take it off and stop pumping, you are right back to where you started. Nevertheless, a pump can be a very stimulating suction toy.

Conclusion

Two hundred questions answered and we have only just begun! After nearly two decades of studying sex I find there is always more to learn. Each individual I encounter has their own unique angle on what is hot, which techniques work best on their body, how they choose to express their sexuality, and how they may structure their relationships. It would impossible to know everything there is to know about sex without meeting every individual who has ever existed. That is part of the joy. Each sex act has the possibility to be an exploration.

If you have more questions, answers, or saucy tales you would like to share with me, please join me online: www.duckydoolittle.com

Finally I would like to say that reading and learning about sex is wonderful but it's all for nothing if you don't take what you learned and do something juicy with it. Get to it and then send me an e-mail and tell me how it goes!

Selected Bibliography

Angier, Natalie. 1999. *Woman: An Intimate Geography*. New York.

Blank, Joani. 1993. *Femalia*. San Francisco.

Blue, Violet. 2002. *The Ultimate Guide to Cunnilingus: How to Go Down on a Woman and Give Her Exquisite Pleasure*. San Francisco.

———. 2002. *The Ultimate Guide to Fellatio: How to Go Down on a Man and Give Him Mind-blowing Pleasure*. San Francisco.

Boston Women's Health Book Collective. 1998. *Our Bodies, Ourselves: For the New Century*. New York.

Carlson, Karen, M.D., Stephanie Eisenstat, M.D., and Terra Ziporyn. 1996. *The Harvard Guide to Women's Health*. Cambridge, Mass.

Chalker, Rebecca. 2000. *The Clitoral Truth: The Secret World at Your Fingertips*. New York.

Chia, Mantak, and Douglas Abrams. 1996. *The Multi-Orgasmic Man: How Any Man Can Experience Multiple Orgasms and Dramatically Enhance His Sexual Relationship*. San Fancisco.

Covington, Stephanie S., Ph.D. 2000. *Awakening Your Sexuality: A Guide for Recovering Women*. Center City, Minn.

dilettopress.org. *Sex Toy Science: Independent Research & Reporting on Sex Toy Science & Technology* August 2003

durex.com. "Global Sex Survey" 2004

The Federation of Feminist Women's Health Center. 1991. *A New View of a Woman's Body*. Los Angeles.

Garbage, Greta. 1999. *That's Disgusting: An Adult Guide to What's Gross, Tasteless, Rude, Crude, and Lewd*. Berkeley.

Govan, A.D.T, C. Hodge, and R. Callander. 1985. *Gynaecology Illustrated.* New York.

Gray, Henry. 1998. *Gray's Anatomy.* New York.

Heiman, Julia R., Ph.D., and Joseph Lopiccolo, Ph.D. 1988. *Becoming Orgasmic: A Sexual and Personal Growth Program for Women.* New York.

Institute for the Advanced Study of Human Sexuality. 1999. *The Complete Guide to Safer Sex.* Fort Lee, N.J.

Joannides, Paul. 2001. *Guide to Getting It On.* Waldport, Oreg.

Johnson, Erica, and Michael Gruzuk. November 28, 2001. *Sex in the Marketplace: Bad Vibrations.* Canadian CBC News report. Kaufman, Miriam, M.D., Cory Silverberg, and Fran Odette. 2003. *The Ultimate Guide to Sex and Disability: For All of Us Who Live with Disabilities, Chronic Pain and Illness.* San Francisco.

Louis, Ron, and David Copeland. 2001. *Sex Lover's Book of Lists.* Paramus, N.J.

Mackay, Judith. 2000. *The Penguin Atlas of Human Sexual Behavior: Sexuality and Sexual Practice Around the World.* New York.

Maines, Rachel P. 1999. *The Technology of Orgasm: "Hysteria," the Vibrator, and Women's Sexual Satisfaction.* Baltimore.

Marazzo, Jeanne, M.D. "STDs & Vaginal Infections in Women Who Have Sex with Women." lesbianstd.com.

Morin, Jack, M.D. 1998. *Anal Pleasure and Health: A Guide for Men and Women.* San Fracisco.

Moser, Charles. 1999. *Health Care Without Shame: A Handbook for the Sexually Diverse and Their Care Givers* San Francisco.

Muscio, Inga. 1998. *Cunt: A Declaration of Independence.* Emeryville, Calif.

Stoppard, Miriam, M.D. 2001. *Women's Health Handbook: What Every Woman Needs to Know About Her Body.* New York.

Venning, Rachel, and Claire Cavanah. 2003. *Sex Toys 101: A Playful Uninhibited Guide.* New York.

wikipedia.org. "Monica Lewinsky."

Winks, Cathy, and Anne Semans. 2002. *The Good Vibrations Guide to Sex.* San Francisco.

Winks, Cathy. 1998. *The Good Vibrations Guide to the G-Spot.* San Francisco.

Resources

Anatomy

Books:

A New View of a Woman's Body, by The Federation of Feminist Women's Health Center (Feminist Health Press, 1991).

Dr. Susan Love's Breast Book, by Susan M. Love (Da Capo, 2005).

The Clitoral Truth: The Secret World at Your Fingertips, by Rebecca Chalker (Seven Stories Press, 2000).

Cunt Coloring Book, by Tee Corinne (Last Gasp, 2001).

Femalia, by Joani Blank (Down There Press, 1993).

The G Spot: And Other Discoveries About Human Sexuality, by Alice Khan Ladas, Beverly Whipple, and John D. Perry (Owl Books, 2005).

The Good Vibrations Guide to the G-spot, by Cathy Winks and Anne Semans (Down There Press, 1998).

Gynaecology Illustrated, by A.D.T. Govan, C. Hodge, and R. Callander (Churchill Livingstone, 1985).

Woman: An Intimate Geography, by Natalie Angier (Anchor Books, 1999).

Web Sites:

Circumcision Information and Resource Pages www.cirp.org
An Internet resource that provides information about all aspects of circumcision.

Erection Photos www.erectionphotos.com
A photo site that displays how truly diverse the male penis can be.

Sex Guides

Books:

Anal Pleasure and Health: A Guide for Men and Women, Third Edition, by Jack Morin, M.D. (Down There Press, 1998).

Becoming Orgasmic: A Sexual and Personal Growth Program for Women, by Julia R. Heiman, Ph.D., and Joseph Lopiccolo, Ph.D. (Simon & Schuster, 1988).

The Big Book of Masturbation: From A to Z, by Martha Cornog (Down There Press, 2003).

The Big O: How to Have Them, Give Them and Keep Them Coming, by Lou Paget (Broadway Books, 2001).

Different Loving: A Complete Exploration of the World of Sexual Dominance and Submission, by Gloria Brame and William Brame (Villard Press, 1996).

The Ethical Slut: A Guide to Infinite Sexual Possibilities, by Dossie Easton and Catherine Liszt (Greenery Press, 1998).

Full Exposure: Opening Up to Sexual Creativity and Erotic Expression, by Bright, Susie (Harper, 2000).

The Good Vibrations Guide to Sex, by Cathy Winks and Anne Semans (Cleis Press, 2002).

The Guide to Getting It On!: The Universe's Coolest and Most Informative Book About Sex, by Paul Joannides (Goofy Foot Press, 2000).

How to Make Great Love to a Woman, by Anne Hooper and Phillip Hodson (Warner Books, 2000).

How to Tell a Naked Man What to Do: Advice from a Woman Who Knows, by Candida Royalle (Fireside, 2004).

The Joy of Cybersex: A Guide for Creative Lovers, by Deb Levine (Ballantine Books, 1998).

Making Love, by Richard Rhodes (Simon & Schuster, 1992).

The Multi-Orgasmic Couple: Sexual Secrets Every Couple Should Know, by Mantak Chia et al. (HarperCollins, 2002).

The Multi-Orgasmic Man, by Mantak Chia and Douglas Abrams (Harper Collins, 1996).

The Penguin Atlas of Human Sexual Behavior: Sexuality and Sexual Practice Around the World, by Judith Mackay (Penguin Reference, 2000).

Position of the Day Playbook: Sex Every Day in Every Way, by Nerve.com (Chronicle Books, 2004).

Screw the Roses, Send Me the Thorns: The Romance and Sexual Sorcery of Sadomasochism, Philip Miller and Molly Devon (Mystic Rose Books, 1995).

Sex for One: The Joy of Self-loving, by Betty Dodson (Harmony, 1987).

Sex Smart: How Your Childhood Shaped Your Sexual Life and What to Do About It, by Aline P. Zoldbrod (New Harbinger Publications, 1998).

She Comes First: The Thinking Man's Guide to Pleasuring a Woman, by Ian Kerner (Regan Books, 2004).

Spectacular Sex: Making Over Your Love Life with One of the World's Greatest Sex Experts, by Annie Sprinkle (Penguin, 2005).

Ultimate Guide to Anal Sex for Women, by Tristan Taormino (Cleis Press, 1997).

The Ultimate Guide to Cunnilingus: How to Go Down on a Woman and Give Her Exquisite Pleasure, by Violet Blue (Cleis Press, 2002).

The Ultimate Guide to Fellatio: How to Go Down on a Man and Give Him Mind-Blowing Pleasure, by Violet Blue (Cleis Press, 2002).

The Ultimate Guide to Sex and Disability: For All of Us Who Live with Disabilities, Chronic Pain and Illness, by Miriam Kaufman, M.D., Cory Silverberg and Fran Odette (Cleis Press, 2003).

The Whole Lesbian Sex Book: A Passionate Guide For All of Us, by Felice Newman (Cleis Press, 1999).

Wild Side Sex: The Book of Kink—Education, Sensual, and Entertaining Essays, by Midori (Daedalus Publishing Company, 2005).

Women's Sexual Passages: Finding Pleasure and Intimacy at Every Stage of Life, by Elizabeth Davis (Hunter House Publishers, 2000).

Web Sites:

Bi Net USA www.binetusa.org

A network of bisexual communities, promoting bisexual visibility, and distributing educational information regarding bisexuality.

Jackin World www.jackinworld.com

The ultimate male masturbation techniques resource and advice site.

Section 12 www.section12.com
A frank and open online community for discussion of intense issues, including BDSM and other forms of kinky sex.

Society for Human Sexuality www.sexuality.org
Hundreds of fantastic articles on sexuality.

Sexuality Information and Education Council of the United States www.siecus.org
Advocates for the right of all people to accurate information, comprehensive education about sexuality, and sexual health services.

Sex Toys

Books:

Sex Toys 101: A Playfully Uninhibited Guide, by Rachel Venning and Claire Cavanah (Simon & Schuster, 2003).

The Technology of Orgasm: "Hysteria," the Vibrator, and Women's Sexual Satisfaction, by Rachel P. Maines (The John Hopkins University Press, 1999).

Online and Boutique Retailers:

A Woman's Touch www.a-womans-touch.com
Adam & Eve www.aeonline.com
Babeland www.babeland.com
Blowfish www.blowfish.com
Coco de Mer www.coco-de-mer.co.uk
Come As Your Are www.comeasyouare.com
Early To Bed www.early2bed.com
Eros Boutique www.erosboutique.org
Eve's Garden www.evesgarden.com
Forbidden Fruit www.forbiddenfruit.com
Glyde Dams www.sheerglydedams.com
Good For Her www.goodforher.com
Good Vibrations www.goodvibes.com

Grand Opening! www.grandopening.com
JT's Stockroom www.stockroom.com
Libida www.libida.com
Liberator Shapes www.liberatorshapes.com
Lovecraft www.lovecraftsexshop.com
O'My Online www.omyonline.com
Pleasure Chest www.thepleasurechest.com
Purple Passion www.purplepassion.com
SH! www.sh-womenstore.com
Smitten Kitten www.smittenkittenonline.com
Vixen Creations www.vixencreations.com
Womyns' Ware www.womynsware.com
X-or www.ilovexor.com
Xandria Collection www.xandria.com

Home Party Retailers:

Athena's Home Novelties www.athenashn.com 1-877-ATHENAS
For Your Pleasure www.foryourpleasure.com 1-888-466-4397
Passion Parties www.passionparties.com 1-800-4-PASSION
Pure Romance www.pureromance.com 1-866-ROMANCE

Erotica and Pornography

Books:

How to Write a Dirty Story: Reading, Writing, and Publishing Erotica, by Susie
    Bright (Fireside, 2002).
My Secret Garden: Women's Sexual Fantasies, by Nancy Friday (Pocketbooks,
    1974).
*The Ultimate Guide to Adult Videos: How to Watch Adult Videos and Make Your Sex
    Life Sizzle,* by Violet Blue (Cleis Press, 2003).

Web Sites:

Adult Video News www.avn.com
    Video reviews and behind the scenes scoop on the adult video business.

Clean Sheets www.cleansheets.com
A weekly magazine devoted to encouraging and publishing quality erotic fiction.

Janes's Guide www.janesguide.com
Honest reviews of sex on the net, from highbrow erotica and fine art nude photography to xxx hardcore.

Literotica www.literotica.com
Original erotic fiction to turn your brain on.

Nerve www.nerve.com
Fearless, intelligent sexuality website for women and men.

On Our Backs www.onourbacksmag.com
The online companion to the honest and hot lesbian porn magazine *On Our Backs*.

Scarlet Letters www.scarletletters.com
Online publishers of humanist, feminist, sex-positive, original erotica.

Sex Educators and Places to Learn

Annie Sprinkle www.anniesprinkle.org
Babeland www.babeland.com
Barbara Carrellas www.barbaracarrellas.com
Betty Dodson www.bettydodson.com
Body Electric www.bodyelectric.org
Candida Royalle www.candidaroyalle.com
Come As Your Are www.comeasyouare.com
Diane Torr www.dianetorr.com
Ducky DooLittle www.duckydoolittle.com
Early To Bed www.early2bed.com
Erotic Massage www.eroticmassage.com
Eulenspiegel Society www.tes.org
Good Vibrations www.goodvibes.com
Grand Opening www.grandopening.com

Kate Bornstein www.katebornstein.com

Lolita www.leatheryenta.com

Lou Paget www.loupaget.com

Midori www.fhp-inc.com

Mistress Morgana www.mistressmorgana.com

Museum of Sex www.mosex.com

Nina Hartley www.nina.com

Sheri Winston www.sheriwinston.com

Smitten Kitten www.smittenkittenonline.com

Tristan Taormino www.puckerup.com

Veronica Vera www.missvera.com

Violet Blue www.tinynibbles.com

Womyns' Ware www.womynsware.com

Body Image and Self-Esteem

Books:

200 Ways to Love the Body You Have, by Marcia Germaine Hutchinson (The Crossing Press, 1999).

Big Big Love: A Sourcebook on Sex for People of Size and Those Who Love Them, by Hanne Blank (Greenery Press, 2000).

Bitches, Bimbos and Ballbreakers: The Guerrilla Girls' Illustrated Guide to Female Stereotypes, by the Guerrilla Girls (Penguin Books, 2003).

Body Outlaws: Young Women Write About Body Image and Identity, by Ophira Edut, ed. (Seal Press, 2000).

Cunt: A Declaration of Independence, by Inga Muscio (Seal Press, 1998).

Exhibitionism for the Shy: Show Off, Dress Up, and Talk Hot, by Carol Queen (Down There Press, 1995).

Fast Girls: Teenage Tribes and the Myth of The Slut, by Emily White (Scribner, 2002).

Looking Queer: Body Image and Identity in Lesbian, Bisexual, Gay, and Transgender Communities, by Dawn Atkins, ed. (Harrington Park Press, 1998).

Nothing to Lose: A Guide to Sane Living in a Larger Body, by Cheri Erdmab (Harper Collins, 1995).

Nymphomania: A History, by Carol Groneman (W. W. Norton & Company, 2000).

Web Sites:

Abundance Magazine www.abundancemagazine.com
> A forum for people of size and their admirers to congregate, to socialize, to exchange ideas and beliefs, and to become familiar with what it is like on the other side of the fence.

Adios Barbie www.adiosbarbie.com
> A body image site for every body.

Fat! So? www.fatso.com
> An online and print magazine for people who don't apologize for their size.

Identity House www.identityhouse.org
> A peer counseling organization of caring volunteers ready to speak with you, listen to you and share the struggles and joys of being gay, lesbian or bisexual or transgender.

Sexual Health

Books:

The African American Woman's Health Book: A Guide to Prevention and Cure of Illness, by Valiere Alcena, M.D. (Barricade Book, 2001).

Awakening Your Sexuality: A Guide for Recovering Women, by Stephanie S. Covington, Ph.D. (Hazelden, 2000).

The Complete Guide to Safer Sex, by the Institute for the Advanced Study of Human Sexuality (Barricade Books, 1999).

Dr. Susan Love's Menopause and Hormone Book: Making Informed Choices, by Susan Love, M.D. (Three Rivers Press, 2003).

The Harvard Guide to Women's Health, by Carlson, Karen, M.D., Stephanie Eisenstat, M.D., and Terra Ziporyn (Harvard University Press, 1996).

Health Care Without Shame: A Handbook For the Sexually Diverse and Their Care Givers, by Charles Moser (Greenery Press 1999).

The Lesbian Health Book: Caring for Ourselves, Jocelyn White, M.D. and Marissa C. Martinez (Seal Press, 1997).

Our Bodies, Ourselves, by Boston Women's Health Book Collective (Touchstone, 1998).

The V Book: A Doctor's Guide to Complete Vulvovaginal Health, Elizabeth Stewart,
M.D. and Paula Spencer (Bantam, 2002).
Women's Health Handbook: What Every Woman Needs to Know About Her Body, by
Miriam Stoppard M.D. (Dorling Kindersley Limited, 2001).

Web Sites:

Alcoholics Anonymous www.alcoholics-anonymous.org

The Body www.thebody.com
A website dedicated to demystifying HIV/AIDS and its treatment for doctors and patients.

Gay Health www.gayhealth.com
Health and wellness site dedicated to lesbian, gay, bisexual and transgender
men and women.

The Gay & Lesbian Medical Association www.glma.org

Feminist Women's Health Centers www.fwhc.org

Guide to Safe & Responsible Sex www.itsyoursexlife.com

Lesbian STD www.lesbiansTD.com
Information and resources regarding sexual health and sexually transmitted
diseases in women who have sex with women.

Luna Pads www.lunapads.com
Responsible products for women's wellness.

Kink Aware Professionals www.bannon.com/kap
A privately funded, nonprofit service dedicated to providing psychotherapeutic,
medical, and legal referrals to professionals who are knowledgeable about and
sensitive to diverse expressions of sexuality.

Sexual Health Network www.sexualhealth.com
Dedicated to providing easy access to sexuality information, education, mutual support, counseling, therapy, health care, products, and other resources for people with disabilities, illness, or natural changes throughout the lifecycle and those who love them or care for them.

Planned Parenthood www.plannedparenthood.org
Provides comprehensive reproductive and complimentary health care services in settings that preserve and protect the essential privacy and rights of each individual. (800) 230-PLAN

WebMD www.webmd.com
Provides valuable health information, tools for managing your health, and support to those who seek information.

Hotlines:
Abortion Hotline (800) 772-9100

Emergency Contraception (800) 584-9911
(888) NOT-2-LATE

Home Access (800) HIV-TEST
HIV at home test.

National AIDS Hotline (800) 342-AIDS
Español (800) 344-7432
Hearing Impaired Access (TTY) (800) 243-7889

National STD Hotline (800) 227-8922

Parenting and Sex

Books:
Changing Bodies, Changing Lives Expanded Third Edition: A Book for Teens on Sex and Relationships, by Ruth Bell (Three Rivers Press, 1998).

Deal with It: A Whole New Approach to Your Body, Brain and Life as a gURL, by
   Esther Drill, Heather McDonald, and Rebecca Odes (Pocket Books, 1999).
*The Hip Mama Survival Guide: Advice from the Trenches on Pregnancy, Childbirth,
   Cool Names, Clueless Doctors, Potty Training and Toddler Avengers,* by Ariel
   Gore (Hypertension Press, 1998).
*No Body's Perfect: Stories by Teens About Body Image, Self-Acceptance and the Search
   for Identity,* by Kirberger, Kimberly (Scholastic Paperbacks, 2003).
Reproductive Issues for People with Disabilities, by Florence P. Haseltine (Paul H.
   Brooke, 1993).
Sexy Mamas: Keeping Your Sex Life Alive While Raising Kids, by Cathy Winks
   and Anne Seman (Inner Ocean Publishing, 2004).
*The Ultimate Guide to Pregnancy for Lesbians: How to Stay Sane and Care for Your-
   self from Pre-conception through Birth,* by Rachel Pepper (Cleis Press, 2005).

Web Sites:
gURL www.gurl.com
   An online community and content site for teenage girls. Very brain, body
   and sex positive.

La Maza www.lamaze.com
   Great section devoted to sex while pregnant and after birth.

Scarleteen www.scarleteen.com
   Sex education for teens and parents.

Surviving Abuse and Nonconsensual Sex

Books:
*Allies in Healing: When the Person You Love Was Sexually Abused As a Child: A
   Support Book,* by Laura Davis (HarperPerennial, 1991).
*Survivor's Guide to Sex: How to Have an Empowered Sex Life after Child Sexual
   Abuse,* by Stacy Haines (Cleis Press, 1999).
The Courage to Heal Workbook: For Women and Men Survivors of Sexual Abuse, by
   Laura Davis (Harper Collins Inc., 1990).

Web Sites:

Rape, Abuse, and Incest National Network www.rainn.org
A free twenty-four-hour hotline for survivors of sexual abuse, rape, and domestic violence. 1-800-656-HOPE

Hotlines:

Childhelp USA National Child Abuse Hotline 1-800-4-A-CHILD
Counselor twenty-four-hour hotline offering crisis intervention information regarding child abuse, resources for survivors, help with parenting, and referrals.

National Domestic Violence Hotline (800) 799-7233

Network for Battered Lesbians and Bisexual Women (617) 423-7233

Survivors of Incest Anonymous (SIA) (410) 282-3400
A twelve-step program—call for groups in your area.